Control of Communicable Diseases in Man

An Official Report of the
American Public Health Association

D0840392

Published by
THE AMERICAN PUBLIC HEALTH ASSOCIATION
1790 Broadway, New York 19, N. Y.

1955

Eighth Edition

This Report has been Approved in Principle by
The United States Public Health Service
and
The Surgeons General of the United States Army,
Navy, and Air Force

The substance of this Report has been accepted by the
Ministry of Health for England and Wales and the Department of Health for Scotland with certain reservations to
meet international commitments and agreements and differences in legislative and administrative practice in Great
Britain.

CONTROL OF COMMUNICABLE DISEASES IN MAN

Preface to the Eighth Edition

THE first edition of this official report of the American Public Health Association was prepared by a committee of the Health Officers Section and published October 12, 1917. In 1935 responsibility for the text passed to the Committee on Research and Standards and revisions by its Subcommittee on Communicable Disease Control have appeared at 5-year intervals. The present eighth edition was prepared by the Subcommittee with the following membership:

John E. Gordon, M.D., Chairman
Gaylord W. Anderson, M.D.
Joseph A. Bell, M.D.
E. Gurney Clark, M.D.
John H. Dingle, M.D.
Donald T. Fraser, M.B.*
William McD. Hammon, M.D.
Robert F. Korns, M.D.

Alexander D. Langmuir, M.D.
Donald S. Martin, M.D.
Henry E. Meleney, M.D.
Ralph S. Muckenfuss, M.D.
Philip E. Sartwell, M.D.
Joseph E. Smadel, M.D.
Franklin H. Top, M.D.

Collaboration was requested by the Committee from the following national and international organizations, which designated their respective representatives:

American Academy of Pediatrics—Aims C. McGuiness, M.D.
Federal Civil Defense Administration—John J. Phair, M.D.
Conference of Public Health Veterinarians—James H. Steele, D.V.M.
Department of the Army—Tom F. Whayne, M.D.
Department of the Navy—James J. Sapero, M.D.
Department of the Air Force—Theodore C. Bedwell, Jr., M.D.
Ministry of Health for England and Wales—G. S. Wilson, M.D.
Department of Health for Scotland—Andrew Davidson, M.D.
Pan American Sanitary Bureau—Carlos Luis González, M.D.
World Health Organization—W. M. Bonné, M.D.

Committee members and consultants took part in exchange of documents and in the meetings of November, 1953 in New York and in Buffalo, New York in 1954, by which common agreement was reached as to the facts and opinions to be presented and the form of their expression. This is the third edition in which the Ministry of Health for England

* Deceased.

1

and Wales and the Department of Health for Scotland have collaborated, and the second in which the World Health Organization has participated.

Purposes of the Manual. The aim is to provide an informative text for ready reference by public health workers of official and voluntary health agencies, to include physicians, dentists, veterinarians, sanitary engineers, public health nurses, social workers, health educators and sanitarians; and for physicians, dentists and veterinarians in private practice having a concern with the control of communicable disease. The booklet is also designed for military physicians and others serving with the armed forces at home and abroad, and for health workers stationed in foreign countries. School administrators, medical students, and students of public health are others finding use for the material presented. The stated aim determines the format of the manual and its pocket size. The booklet does not substitute for standard text books. To meet the defined uses, the content is broadly representative of global infectious disease. While primarily intended for workers in the Americas and therefore largely expressive of American practices and ideas, a wider usefulness of the publication is seen in its translation into French, German, Spanish, Portuguese, Serbo-Croatian, Japanese, Chinese, Thai and Finnish.

A second general purpose is to serve public health administrators as a guide and as a source of materials in preparation of regulations and legal requirements for the control of the communicable diseases, in development of programs for health education of the public, and in the administrative acts of official health agencies toward management of communicable disease. The needs of field workers have had attention through inclusion of much information applicable to field operations, primarily methods of control as they relate to preventive measures, to control of the infected individual, contacts and environment, and to management of epidemics.

The intent is to present factual knowledge in brief fashion and to advance opinion consistent with those facts as a basis for intelligent management of communicable disease, unhampered by local usage and not restricted to prevailing practices. Recommendations towards standard administrative or technical procedure are avoided, because local conditions and interrelated problems commonly require variation from state to state within the United States, and between countries. The emphasis is on principle, because variations in practice are also due to incomplete knowledge of recent advances and of successful practices under other and similar conditions. Attempt is made to keep facts and opinions current by periodic revision of the manual.

Scope and Content. The report originally was designed as an aid in formulating standard regulations for administrative control of communicable diseases for which notification was usually required by state and municipal health authorities of the United States. Subsequently the content was enlarged to include diseases of South America, and eventually some of the more important infections wholly outside the Western Hemisphere. Largely because of overseas military activities, this feature was expanded in the 5th and 6th editions. Because of increasing international health activities in which many American workers participate, decision was taken that the 8th edition give more comprehensive coverage of world infections. The list is by no means complete, but most conditions of public health importance are included, with a goodly representation of the less common and less significant which so often present puzzling problems. The 7th edition had descriptions of 92 diseases, the 8th edition has 118. Presentation of infections due to fungi, spirochetes, protozoa and helminths has been materially strengthened.

Modern methods of antibiotic treatment and chemotherapy have become a significant feature of control procedures by limiting periods of communicability and thus decreasing community dosage of infectious agents. This is aside from their value in reducing fatality and mortality. The present edition therefore presents more detailed information on specific methods of management of infected persons.

The index is much enlarged. An added feature is the collection of references to various diseases according to sources of infection, reservoirs, common vehicles and vectors involved in transmission, measures against arthropods, methods for active and passive immunization, and for chemoprophylaxis.

As in earlier editions, the terms used are first defined. Each disease is briefly identified, with regard to clinical nature, laboratory diagnosis and differentiation of allied or related conditions. Etiologic agent, source and reservoir of infection, mode of transmission, incubation period, period of communicability, susceptibility and resistance, and occurrence are next presented. Following this are described methods of control under the following four headings.

A. *Preventive Measures:* Applicable generally to individuals and groups when and where the particular disease may occur in sporadic, epidemic, or endemic form, whether or not the disease is an active threat at the moment, e.g., vaccination against smallpox, chlorination of water supplies, pasteurization of milk, control of rodents and arthropods, animal control, and immunization.

B. *Control of the Infected Individual, Contacts, and Environment:* Those measures designed to prevent infectious matter present in the person and environment of the infected individual from being conveyed to other persons, arthropods or animals in a way to spread the disease, and to keep contacts under surveillance during the assumed period of incubation of the disease and carriers under control until they are found to be free of infecting agents of the disease in question.   Specific treatment is included under this heading and represents opinion as of 1955.

C. *Epidemic Measures:* Those procedures of emergency character designed to limit the spread of a communicable disease which has developed widely in a group or community or within an area, state, or nation, such measures being unnecessary or not justified when the disease occurs sporadically or separated by considerable intervals in time, and only among widely separated individuals.

D. *International Measures:* Such controls of population movements, commerce, and transportation of immigrants and travellers across national boundaries as may arise from international sanitary regulations or result from conferences or agreements between governments and give promise of protection of uninfected populations in one or more nations against the known and notified risk of infection from another nation where the particular disease in question may be present in endemic or epidemic form. Vaccination and other immunization precautions, and quarantine and surveillance of travellers are included, also animal control and immunization.

Reporting of Communicable Disease. Notification to the local health authority that a case of communicable disease exists within the particular jurisdiction is the first step toward control. Administrative practice as to what diseases are to be reported and how they should be reported varies greatly from one region to another. This is justified in part by different conditions and different frequencies of disease. The present edition of this manual presents a basic scheme of reporting, directed toward practical working procedure rather than ideal practice, and uninhibited by tradition of what is now done. The purpose is encouragement and uniformity of morbidity reporting, to permit comparability of data within this country and between nations.

A system of reporting functions at four levels. The first is collection of the basic data in the local community where disease occurs. The data are next assembled at district, state or provincial level. The third step is the collection of total information under national auspices. Finally, for certain prescribed diseases report is made by the national health authority to the World Health Organization.

Adequate control of communicable disease requires action at all four levels, for each jurisdictional authority has its prescribed responsibilities for application and development of necessary measures. To function effectively, each needs an exchange of current information on disease frequencies, which is accomplished through forwarding data collected at the local level, and summarization and return report by higher jurisdiction. The local health authority is thus informed of prevailing disease in its own particular area, in areas from which disease may invade, and is in position to make use of the extensive knowledge and facilities available in the whole health organization.

Consideration is here limited to the first stage of a reporting system, the collection of the basic data at local level; first because that is the fundamental part of any scheme, and second because this manual is primarily for local health workers. The basic data sought at local level are of two kinds (Definition 27, Report of a Disease, p. 16).

1. Report of Cases. Each local health authority, in conformity with regulations of higher authority, will determine what diseases are to be reported as a routine and regular procedure, who is responsible for reporting, the nature of the report required and the manner in which reports are forwarded to the next superior jurisdiction.

Physicians are required to report all notifiable illnesses which come to their attention; in addition, the statutes or regulations of many localities require reporting by hospital, householder or other person having knowledge of a case of a reportable disease.

Case Report of a communicable disease provides minimal identifying data of name, address, diagnosis, age, sex, and date of report for each patient and in some instances for suspects; dates of onset and of diagnosis are useful.

Collective Report is the assembled number of cases by diagnosis occurring within a prescribed time and without individual identifying data, e.g. 20 cases of malaria, week ending Oct. 6.

2. Report of Epidemics. In addition to requirement of individual case report, any unusual or group expression of illness which may be of public concern (Definition 11, Epidemic, p. 14) is desirably reported to the local health authority by the most expeditious means, whether well known and subject to routine report, indefinite or unknown, or absent from the list of diseases officially reportable in the particular locality. Pertinent data of the Epidemic Report include number of cases, within what time, approximate population involved, and apparent mode of spread. The report is forwarded to next superior jurisdiction by telephone or telegraph.

Aside from the recommended requirement on Report of Epidemics, just stated, the communicable diseases listed in this manual are distributed among the following five classes, according to desirability and practical benefit presumably to be derived from reporting. These classes are referred to by number throughout the text, under Section 9B1 of each disease. The purpose is to provide a basis by which each health jurisdiction may determine its list of regularly reportable diseases.

Class 1. *Case Report Universally Required by International Sanitary Regulation*

This class is limited to the six internationally quarantinable diseases, which are cholera, plague, louse-borne relapsing fever, smallpox, louse-borne typhus fever and yellow fever.

Obligatory case report to local health authority by telephone, telegraph or other rapid means. The local health authority forwards the report to next superior jurisdiction by similar method if it is the first recognized case in the local area, or the first case outside those limits of the local area already affected; otherwise weekly by mail, or telegraphically in unusual situations.

Class 2. *Case Report Regularly Required Wherever the Disease Occurs*

Two subclasses are recognized, based on relative urgency for investigation of contacts and source of infection, or for starting control measures.

A. Case report by telephone, telegraph or other rapid means; forward to next superior jurisdiction weekly by mail, except that first recognized case in territory or first case outside limits of local area already affected is by telegraph; examples, typhoid fever, diphtheria.

B. Case report by most practicable means; forward to next superior jurisdiction as a collective report, weekly by mail; examples, brucellosis, leprosy.

Class 3. *Selectively Reportable in Recognized Endemic Areas*

In many states and countries, diseases of this class are not reportable. Reporting may be prescribed in particular regions, states or countries by reason of undue frequency or severity. Where applicable to the United States, USA is specified after "endemic areas." Three subclasses are recognized; A and B are primarily useful under conditions of established endemicity as a means toward prompt control measures and to judge effectiveness of control programs; the main purpose of C is to stimulate control measures or to acquire essential epidemiological data.

A. Case report by telephone, telegraph or other rapid means in specified areas where the disease ranks in importance with Class 2A; not reportable in many countries; examples, tularemia, scrub typhus.

B. Case report by most practicable means; forwarded to next superior jurisdiction as a collective report by mail weekly or monthly; not reportable in many countries; examples, Bartonellosis, coccidioidomycosis.

C. Collective report weekly by mail to local health authority; forward to next superior jurisdiction by mail weekly, monthly, quarterly or sometimes annually; examples, clonorchiasis, phlebotomus fever.

Class 4. *Obligatory Report of Epidemics; No Case Report Required*

Prompt report of outbreaks of particular public health importance by telephone, telegraph or other rapid means; forward to next superior jurisdiction by telephone or telegraph. Pertinent data include number of cases, within what time, approximate population involved, and apparent mode of spread; examples, food poisoning, influenza.

Class 5. *Official Report Not Ordinarily Justifiable*

Diseases of this class are of two general kinds: those typically sporadic and uncommon, often not directly transmissible from man to man; or of such epidemiological nature as to offer no practical measures for control; examples, blastomycosis, common cold.

Diseases are often made reportable although the information gathered is put to no practical use. This frequently has the result that the general level of reporting deteriorates, even for diseases of much importance. Better case reporting is usually to be had by restricting official report to those diseases for which control services are provided, or potential control procedures are under evaluation, or epidemiological information is needed for a definite purpose.

Acknowledgments. Grateful acknowledgment is made for expert opinion and critical comment received from many physicians and others, both within and without the Association. Many colleagues from other countries have contributed to the accuracy and completeness of the report, especially through personal experience in research and control of infections absent or not commonly present in the United States. Diseases common to animals and man have had the benefit of veterinary opinion. The final acknowledgment is fittingly reserved for Haven Emerson, M.D.; he originated this manual and directed its activities throughout its history, including the 1950 revision. In the preparation of this 8th edition he has been a most industrious unofficial consultant.

TABLE OF CONTENTS

9

12 TABLE OF CONTENTS

DEFINITIONS

(Technical meaning of terms used in the text)

1. *Animal host.*—An animal other than man which under natural conditions harbors an infectious agent pathogenic for man.

2. *Carrier.*—A carrier is a person who harbors a specific infectious agent in the absence of discernible clinical disease and serves as a potential source or reservoir of infection for man. The carrier state may occur with infections inapparent throughout their course (commonly known as healthy carriers), and also as a feature of incubation period, convalescence and post-convalescence of infections having a recognized clinical stage (commonly known as incubatory and convalescent carriers). Under either circumstance the carrier state may be short or long (temporary or chronic carriers). The same applies to animal carriers.

3. *Cleaning.*—The removal from surfaces by scrubbing and washing, as with hot water, soap, and washing soda (Na_2CO_3) or other detergent, of infectious agents and organic matter on which and in which infectious agents may find favorable conditions for prolonging life and virulence.

4. *Communicable disease.*—An illness due to an infectious agent or its toxic products which is transmitted directly or indirectly to a well person from an infected person or animal, or through the agency of an intermediate animal host, vector, or the inanimate environment. This report also includes infestations by ectoparasites such as pediculosis. (See 20, Infestation.)

5. *Communicable period.*—The time or times during which the etiologic agent may be transferred directly or indirectly from an infected person to another person, or from an infected animal to man.

In diseases such as diphtheria and scarlet fever, in which mucous membranes are involved from the first entry of the pathogen, the period of communicability is from the date of first exposure to a source of infection, until the infecting microorganism is no longer disseminated from the involved mucous membranes; i.e., from before the prodromata until the termination of a carrier state, if such develops.

In diseases such as tuberculosis, syphilis, and gonorrhea, the communicable state may be at any time over a long and sometimes intermittent period when unhealed lesions of the disease permit the discharge of infectious agents from the surface of the skin or through any of the body orifices. In certain diseases communicability does not occur during the early incubation period or after full recovery; e.g., measles and chickenpox.

In diseases transmitted by arthropods, such as malaria and yellow fever, the periods of communicability are those during which the etiologic agent occurs in the blood or other tissues of the infected person in infective form and in sufficient numbers for vector infection. A period of communicability is also to be distinguished for the arthropod, namely that time during which the agent is present in the tissues of the arthropod in such form as to be capable of transmitting infection.

6. *Contact.*—A contact is any person or animal known to have been in such association with an infected person or animal as to have had the opportunity of acquiring the infection. Contact may be immediate and intimate, involving touching or close approximation of sick and well; or remote or casual with no direct physical contact. Familial contacts are those living within the household of an infected person, as distinguished from those where contact came through work, school or play.

7. *Contamination.*—The presence of a pathogenic agent on a body surface or on or in an inanimate article or substance.

8. *Disinfection.*—Killing of pathogenic agents outside the body by chemical or physical means directly applied.

Concurrent disinfection is the application of disinfection as soon as possible after the discharge of infectious material from the body of an infected person, or after the soiling of articles with such infectious discharges, all personal contact with such discharges or articles being prevented prior to such disinfection.

Terminal disinfection indicates the process of rendering the personal clothing and immediate physical environment of the patient free from the possibility of conveying the infection to others, after the patient has been removed, or has ceased to be a source of infection or after isolation practices have been discontinued.

9. *Disinfestation.*—Any physical or chemical process serving to destroy undesired animal forms, especially arthropods or rodents, present upon the person, the clothing, or in the environment of an individual, or on domestic animals. (See 21, Insecticide and 30, Rodenticide infra.) This includes the processes commonly called "delousing" as applied to infestation with Pediculus humanus, the body louse.

10. *Education in personal cleanliness.*—This phrase includes the various means available to impress upon all members of the community, young and old, and especially when communicable disease is prevalent or during epidemics, by spoken and printed word, and by illustration and suggestion, the necessity of :

    a. Keeping the body clean by sufficiently frequent soap and water baths.

    b. Washing hands in soap and water immediately after voiding bowels or bladder and always before eating.

    c. Keeping hands and unclean articles, or articles that have been used for toilet purposes by others, away from the mouth, nose, eyes, ears, genitalia, and wounds.

    d. Avoiding the use of common or unclean eating, drinking, or toilet articles of any kind, such as cutlery and crockery, drinking cups, towels, handkerchiefs, combs, hairbrushes, and pipes.

    e. Avoiding exposure of persons to spray from the nose and mouth, as in coughing, sneezing, laughing, or talking.

    f. Washing hands thoroughly after handling the patient or his belongings and wearing a protective overall apron while in the sickroom.

11. *Epidemic.*—An epidemic or outbreak is here defined as the occurrence in a community or region of a group of illnesses of similar nature, clearly in excess of normal expectancy, and derived from a common or propagated source. The number of cases indicating presence of an epidemic will vary according to the etiologic agent, size and type of population exposed, previous experience or lack of exposure to the disease, and time and place of occurrence; epidemicity is thus relative to usual frequency of the disease in the same area, among the specified population, at the same season of year. A single case of a communicable disease long absent from a population or first invasion by a disease not previously recognized in that area is to be considered as a potential epidemic and meeting the requirements in respect to reporting of epidemics, as dengue fever in Florida or American trypanosomiasis in Texas.

12. *Fumigation.*—Any process by which the killing of animal forms, especially arthropods and rodents, is accomplished by the employment of gaseous agents. (See 21, Insecticide and 30, Rodenticide.)

13. *Immune person.*—An immune person is one who possesses specific protective antibodies or cellular immunity as a result of previous infection or immunization, or is so conditioned by such previous specific experience as to respond adequately with production of antibodies sufficient in either instance to protect from illness following exposure to the etiologic agent of the disease. This applies also to animals. Immunity is relative; an ordinarily effective protection may be overwhelmed by an excessive dose of the infectious agent or an unusual portal of entry.

14. *Inapparent infection.*—A person or animal has an inapparent infection (also known as latent or subclinical infection) when the infectious agent has so mild an effect that even though infection be present and is identifiable by laboratory means, it is undetected clinically.

15. *Incidence.*—The number of cases of disease, of infection or other event occurring during a prescribed time period, in relation to the unit of population in which they occur (a dynamic measurement); thus the incidence of tuberculosis expressed as a rate is the number of new cases reported per 100,000 population per year.

16. *Incubation period.*—The time interval between the infection of a susceptible person or animal and the appearance of signs or symptoms of the disease in question.

17. *Infected person.*—Infected persons include patients or sick persons, persons with inapparent infection, and carriers. The same expression holds for animals, including arthropods.

18. *Infection.*—The entry and development or multiplication of a particular pathogen in the body of man or animal. The presence of living infectious agents on exterior surfaces of the body or upon articles of apparel or toilet articles, is not infection but contamination of such surfaces and articles. The term "infection" should not be used to describe conditions of inanimate matter such as soil, water, sewage, milk, or food; the term "contamination" applies (see 7, Contamination).

19. *Infectious disease.*—A disease of man or animal resulting from an infection.

20. *Infestation.*—By infestation of persons and animals is meant the lodgment, development, and reproduction of arthropods on the surface of the body or in the clothing. Infested articles or premises are such as harbor or give shelter to animal forms, especially arthropods and rodents.

21. *Insecticide.*—Any chemical substance used for the destruction of arthropods, whether applied as powder, liquid, atomized liquid, aerosol, or as a paint-spray with residual action. The term larvicide is generally used to designate insecticides applied specifically for destruction of immature stages of arthropods; imagocide and adulticide to designate those applied to destroy mature and adult forms.

22. *Isolation.*—The separation for the period of communicability of infected persons from other persons, in such places and under such conditions as will prevent the direct or indirect conveyance of the infectious agent from infected persons to other persons who are susceptible or who may spread the agent to others. This applies also to animals.

Strict isolation of the patient for the period of communicability is necessary in certain diseases, notably smallpox. However, isolation of the patient has but little effect in limiting the spread of many other diseases, for instance poliomyelitis.

When used in connection with such diseases as the common cold, influenza, chickenpox, mumps, and the pneumonias, isolation is not to be understood, under ordinary circumstances, as a necessary or practicable procedure for official requirement or enforcement, but a modified practice to be instituted under the direction of the attending physician, and its duration to be generally, if not exclusively, at his discretion.

Other than for rare exceptions and under special circumstances, the placarding of premises has no place in public health practice as a means to enforce isolation.

23. *Patient or sick person.*—A person suffering from a recognizable attack of a communicable disease.

24. *Prevalence.*—The number of cases of disease, of infected persons, or of persons with some other attribute, present at a particular time and in relation to the size of the population from which drawn (a static measurement); thus the prevalence of tuberculosis is commonly expressed as the number of active cases (all forms, old and new) existing at a designated time per 100,000 persons.

25. *Quarantine.*—(1) Complete quarantine is the limitation of freedom of movement of such well persons or domestic animals as have been exposed to a communicable disease, for a period of time equal to the longest usual incubation period of the disease, in such manner as to prevent effective contact with those not so exposed.

(2) Modified quarantine is a selective, partial limitation of freedom of movement of persons or domestic animals, commonly on the basis of known or presumed differences in susceptibility, but sometimes because of danger of disease transmission. It may be designed to meet particular situations; examples are exclusion of children from school or exemption of immune persons from provisions required of susceptible persons, prohibition of contacts from acting as food handlers, or restriction of military populations to the post or to quarters.

(3) Surveillance is the practice of close supervision of contacts for purposes of prompt recognition of infection or illness but without restricting their movements.

(4) Segregation is the separation for special consideration, control, or observation of some part of a group of persons or of domestic animals from the others, to facilitate the control of a communicable disease. Removal of susceptible children to homes of immune persons, or the establishment of a sanitary boundary to protect uninfected from infected portions of a population are examples.

26. *Repellent.*—A chemical applied to the skin or clothing or other places to discourage arthropods from lighting on and attacking an individual who cannot be protected otherwise.

27. *Report of a disease.*—Official report is notification of the occurrence of a communicable or other disease in man or animals; to the local health authority for diseases of man, to the livestock, sanitary or agriculture authority for diseases of animals, and in some instances, disease of both animal and man to the health authority. Report should include suspect cases of diseases of particular public health importance, ordinarily those requiring epidemiologic investigation or initiation of special control measures.

When a person is infected in one health jurisdiction and the case is reported from another, the authority receiving the report should notify the other jurisdiction involved, especially if the disease is such as to require examination of contacts for infection, and of food or water supplies as vehicles.

In addition to routine reporting of specified diseases, as determined by the needs of the particular health jurisdiction, special notification of all epidemics or outbreaks of disease, including those not in the list declared reportable, is regularly to be required (see 11, Epidemic).

28. *Reservoir of Infection.*—Reservoirs of infection are man, animals, plants, soil, or inanimate organic matter, in which an infectious agent lives and multiplies and depends primarily for survival, reproducing itself in such manner that it can be transmitted to man. Man himself is the most frequent reservoir of infectious agents pathogenic for man.

29. *Resistance.*—The sum total of body mechanisms which interpose barriers to the progress of invasion of infectious agents.

   a. Immunity—Immunity is here defined as that resistance usually associated with possession of antibodies for a specific disease. Passive immunity is attained either naturally by maternal transfer, or artificially by inoculation of specific protective antibodies (convalescent or immune serum, or gamma globulin) and is of brief duration. Active immunity is attained either naturally by infection, with or without clinical manifestations, or artificially by inoculation of fractions or products of the infectious agent, or of the agent itself in killed, modified or variant form.

   b. Inherent insusceptibility—Inherent insusceptibility is an ability to resist disease independently of antibodies or specifically developed tissue response; it commonly rests in anatomic or physiologic characteristics of the host; it may be genetic or acquired; permanent or temporary; autarcesis.

30. *Rodenticide.*—A chemical substance used for the destruction of rodents, generally through ingestion. (Compare 12, Fumigation.)

31. *Source of Infection.*—The thing, person, object or substance from which an infectious agent passes immediately to a host. Transfer is often direct from reservoir to host in which case the reservoir is also the source of infection (measles). The source may be at any point in the chain of transmission, as a vehicle, vector, intermediate animal host or fomite; thus, contaminated water (typhoid), an infective mosquito (yellow fever), beef (tapeworm infection), or a toy (diphtheria). In each instance cited the reservoir is an infected person. (Compare 28, Reservoir.)

32. *Susceptible.*—A person or animal presumably not possessing resistance against a particular pathogenic agent and for that reason liable to contract a disease if exposed to such agent.

33. *Suspect.*—A person whose medical history and symptoms suggest that he may have or be developing some communicable disease.

34. *Transmission of infection.*—Modes of transmission are the mechanisms by which an infectious agent is transported from reservoir to susceptible human host. They are:

   a. Contact:
      (1) Direct contact: Actual touching of the infected person or animal or other reservoir of infection, as in kissing, sexual intercourse or other contiguous personal association.
      (2) Indirect contact: Touching of contaminated objects such as toys, handkerchiefs, soiled clothing, bedding, surgical instruments and dressings, with subsequent hand to mouth transfer; less commonly, transfer to abraded or intact skin or mucous membrane.

    (3) Droplet spread: The projection on to the conjunctivae and the face or into the nose or mouth of the spray emanating from an infected person during sneezing, coughing, singing or talking. Such droplets usually travel not more than 3 feet from the source. Transmission by droplet infection is considered a form of contact infection, since it involves reasonably close association between two or more persons.

b. Vehicle: Water, food, milk, biological products to include serum and plasma, or any substance or article serving as an intermediate means by which the infectious agent is transported from a reservoir and introduced into a susceptible host through ingestion, through inoculation or by deposit on skin or mucous membrane.

c. Vector: Arthropods or other invertebrates which transmit infection by inoculation into or through the skin or mucous membrane by biting, or by deposit of infective materials on the skin or on food or other objects. The vector may be infected itself or may act only as a passive or mechanical carrier of the agent.

d. Air Borne:

    (1) Droplet nuclei: The inhalation of the small residues which result from evaporation of droplets (see a(3) above) and remain suspended in air of enclosed spaces for relatively long periods of time. Droplet nuclei also may be created purposely by a variety of atomizing devices, or accidentally in the course of many laboratory procedures.

    (2) Dust: The inhalation or settling on body surfaces of coarser particles which may arise from contaminated floors, clothes, bedding, or soil, and ordinarily remain suspended in the air for relatively short periods of time.

ACTINOMYCOSIS

1. *Identification.*—A chronic suppurative or granulomatous process, most frequently localized in jaw, lungs or abdomen, and characterized by swellings, firm at first but later breaking down to form multiple draining sinuses. The course is long and recovery uncommon, with death usually from some intercurrent disease.

   Naked eye or hand lens examination of materials from lesions or discharges usually shows small "sulfur granules" which microscopic examination identifies as actual colonies of the fungus; diagnosis confirmed by anaerobic culture of the fungus.

2. *Etiologic agent.*—Actinomyces bovis (Actinomyces israeli).

3. *Source and reservoir of infection.*—The source of clinical infection is the oral cavity of man where the fungus maintains an inapparent infection around carious teeth and in tonsillar crypts; reservoir unknown.

4. *Mode of transmission.*—From the site of inapparent infection in the mouth, the fungus may be swallowed, inhaled or introduced into jaw tissues by injury. Not known to be transmissible in nature from man to man or from animal to animal.

5. *Incubation period.*—Unknown; probably weeks or months.

6. *Period of communicability.*—Contamination of the environment as long as infection persists; a chronic disease.

7. *Susceptibility and resistance.*—Natural susceptibility is low. No immunity follows attack.

8. *Occurrence.*—An infrequent disease of man, occurring sporadically all over the world. All races, both sexes and all age groups may be affected; the ratio of males to females is approximately two to one, and most cases are between ages 15 and 35. Primarily a disease of cattle, swine, horses and other animals.

9. *Methods of control:*

   A. Preventive measures: Meat inspection of slaughtered animals, with condemning of affected parts, is commonly required by law.

   B. Control of the infected individual, contacts and environment:
      1. Report to local health authority: Official report not ordinarily justifiable, Class 5 (p. 7).
      2. Isolation: None.
      3. Concurrent disinfection: Of discharges and contaminated dressings.
      4. Terminal disinfection: Thorough cleaning.
      5. Quarantine: None.
      6. Immunization: None.
      7. Investigation of contacts and source of infection: Not profitable.
      8. Specific treatment: Prolonged administration of sulfonamides, penicillin, chlortetracycline (aureomycin) or chloramphenicol.

   C. Epidemic measures: Not applicable, a sporadic disease.

   D. International measures: None.

AFRICAN TICK–BORNE FEVER, RICKETTSIAL

1. *Identification.*—A mild to moderately severe illness, characterized by an initial lesion, called the "tache noir" in boutonneuse fever, a febrile period of a few days to two weeks and a generalized maculopapular erythematous rash which appears about the fourth or fifth day and usually involves palms and soles. Although the initial lesion heals slowly, often leaving a scar, the fever and generalized rash seldom persist more than 6 to 7 days. The fatality is less than 3%, even without specific therapy. Synonyms: Boutonneuse Fever, South African Tick-bite Fever, Mediterranean Fever.

    Laboratory diagnosis is by animal inoculation or through demonstrating antibodies by serologic test using a specific rickettsial antigen. The Weil-Felix test (reaction with Proteus OX 19) is frequently positive but the end titer is usually lower than in other rickettsial diseases.

2. *Etiologic agent.*—Rickettsia conorii, a member of the spotted fever group of rickettsiae.

3. *Source and reservoir of infection.*—Infected ticks are the immediate source of infection; whether the reservoir is tick or animal host, or both, is indeterminate.

4. *Mode of transmission.*—In the Mediterranean area, by bite of infected Rhipicephalus sanguineus which infests dogs and their habitations. In South Africa a number of ticks are infected in nature and presumed to be vectors, viz., Haemaphysalis leachi, Amblyomma hebraeum, Rhipicephalus appendiculatus, Boophilus decoloratus and Hyaloma aegyptium.

5. *Incubation period.*—Average 5 to 6 days.

6. *Period of communicability.*—Not communicable from man to man. Ticks remain infectious for life, commonly as long as 18 months; transovarian infection occurs.

7. *Susceptibility and resistance.*—Susceptibility appears to be general and one attack confers immunity.

8. *Occurrence.*—In the Mediterranean and Black Sea areas and widely throughout Africa but not in the Western Hemisphere. In more temperate areas the highest incidence is during warmer months when ticks are prevalent; in tropical areas throughout the year. Outbreaks may occur when groups of susceptibles are brought into an endemic area.

9. *Methods of control:*

    A. Preventive measures:

    1. Personal prophylaxis is by avoiding tick infested areas when feasible, or by taking precautions to prevent tick bite including application of newer tick repellents, or by prompt removal of attached ticks without crushing and without contaminating the hands.
    2. Attempts to reduce numbers of ticks in nature is generally impractical but in areas where the dog and R. sanguineus are important members of the cycle, local measures are indicated, including stray dog control.
    3. Vaccines are not available commercially.

B. Control of the infected individual, contacts and environment:
   1. Report to local health authority: In selected endemic areas; in many countries not a reportable disease. Class 3 B (p. 7).
   2. Isolation: None.
   3. Concurrent disinfection: None.
   4. Terminal disinfection: None.
   5. Quarantine: None.
   6. Immunization: None.
   7. Investigation of contacts and source of infection: Pest control measures against ticks infesting households and dogs.
   8. Specific treatment: One of the tetracycline antibiotics, or chloramphenicol orally until afebrile (about two days) and for one additional day.

C. Epidemic measures: Rarely required; general application of measures listed under 9A1 and 2, careful observation of group at risk with prompt antibiotic therapy for those becoming ill, disinfestation of selected terrain by insecticides (see Rocky Mountain Spotted Fever, p. 157).

D. International measures: Effort to prevent introduction of infected ticks and their vertebrate hosts into areas believed free of the disease.

ANCYLOSTOMIASIS

1. *Identification.*—A chronic debilitating infection with nematodes, commonly known as hookworms. A variety of vague symptoms occur, varying greatly according to degree of infection. The blood-sucking activity of the worms and a predisposing malnutrition lead to hypochromic microcytic anemia. Infected children may be retarded in mental and physical development. Death is infrequent either in acute or chronic stages, and then usually in association with other infection. Synonyms: Uncinariasis, Hookworm Disease.

   Hookworm infection is confirmed by finding the eggs in feces; species recognition is through microscopic examination of adult worms.

2. *Etiologic agent.*—Necator americanus and Ancylostoma duodenale. Third-stage larvae pass from the skin via lymphatics and blood stream to the lungs, enter the alveoli, migrate up the trachea to the pharynx, are swallowed, and reach the small intestine where they attach to the intestinal wall, develop to maturity and produce eggs.

   Infective larvae of cat and dog hookworm (Ancylostoma braziliense and A. caninum) cause a dermatitis in man called creeping eruption; the larvae are destroyed in the skin and do not otherwise affect man.

3. *Source and reservoir of infection.*—The usual source of infection is soil contaminated with infective larvae. Reservoir is feces of infected persons.

4. *Mode of transmission.*—Eggs in feces are deposited on the ground, hatch, larvae develop to the third stage (infective form) and penetrate the skin, usually the foot, in so doing characteristically producing a dermatitis (ground itch). Infection via the alimentary tract is also possible.

5. *Incubation period.*—The first eggs appear in the feces about six weeks after infection. Symptoms may appear after a few weeks to many months or even years, depending on intensity of infection.

6. *Period of communicability.*—Infected individuals are potential spreaders of infection as long as they remain infected and continue to pollute soil, often many years. Under favorable conditions, third-stage infective larvae remain alive in soil for several weeks.

7. *Susceptibility and resistance.*—Susceptibility is universal but the disease is less frequent among Negroes than whites. Some immunity develops with infection.

8. *Occurrence.*—Widely endemic in those tropical and subtropical countries where disposal of feces is inadequate, and soil, moisture, and temperature favor development of infective larvae. N. americanus is the prevailing species throughout tropical West Africa and southeastern United States; and A. duodenale in Mediterranean countries, including the Nile valley. Both forms occur in many parts of Asia, South America and the West Indies.

9. *Methods of control:*

A. Preventive measures:
1. Education as to dangers of soil pollution and methods of prevention.
2. Prevention of soil pollution by installation of sanitary disposal systems for human discharges, especially sanitary privies in rural areas, and education of the public in the use of such facilities.
3. Personal prophylaxis by cleanliness and the wearing of shoes.

B. Control of the infected individual, contacts and environment:
1. Report to local health authority: In selected endemic areas (USA); in most countries not a reportable disease. Class 3C (p. 7).
2. Isolation: None.
3. Concurrent disinfection: Sanitary disposal of feces to prevent contamination of soil and water.
4. Terminal disinfection: None.
5. Quarantine: None.
6. Immunization: None.
7. Investigation of contacts and source of infection: Each patient and carrier is a potential or actual spreader of the disease. Examine all family contacts.
8. Specific treatment: Tetrachlorethylene or hexylresorcinol; toxic reactions are infrequent and therapy can be repeated if necessary. The duration of communicability is shortened.

C. Epidemic measures: Surveys for prevalence in highly endemic areas, public health education in sanitation of the environment and in personal hygiene, and provision of facilities for treatment.

D. International measures: None.

ANTHRAX

1. *Identification.*—An acute bacterial infection of animals and man; in man usually a disease of the skin. An initial papule and vesicle at the site of inoculation turns into an eschar, followed by hard edematous swelling of deeper and adjacent tissues. Pain in the early stages is unusual. If untreated, infection extends progressively to regional lymph nodes and blood stream and may result in overwhelming septicemia and death. Primary anthrax pneumonia and primary gastro-intestinal anthrax are rare. Untreated cutaneous anthrax has a fatality of about 20%; other forms are highly fatal; appreciably lower rates with effective antibiotic therapy. Synonym: Malignant Pustule.

   Laboratory confirmation is by inoculation of mice with exudates from lesions or with blood or other tissues; also by direct demonstration of bacilli in lesions or discharges, and by culture.

2. *Etiologic agent.*—Bacillus anthracis.

3. *Source and reservoir of infection.*—The source of infection is the tissues of animals dying of the disease, or contaminated hair, wool and hides. The reservoir is any one of several species of herbivorous animals, cattle, sheep, goats, horses, and others.

4. *Mode of transmission.*—Infection of skin is by common vehicles (fomites), hair, wool, hides, contaminated shaving brushes and other manufactured products, or by direct contact with infected tissues. Primary anthrax pneumonia when it occurs, presumably results from inhalation of spores. Gastro-intestinal anthrax results from ingestion of heavily contaminated meat; milk is not involved. The disease spreads among herbivorous animals through contaminated soil or feed, and among omnivorous and carnivorous animals through contaminated meat, bone meal or other feed products. Flies may serve as mechanical carriers. Vultures have spread the infection from one area to another. Accidental infections occur among laboratory workers.

5. *Incubation period.*—Within 7 days, usually less than 4.

6. *Period of communicability.*—Rarely if ever transmitted from man to man, although discharges from lesions are infective. Contaminated articles and soil may remain infective for years.

7. *Susceptibility and resistance.*—Uncertain.

8. *Occurrence.*—Infrequent and sporadic in man, primarily as an occupational hazard to veterinarians and agricultural workers handling animals, and to industrial workers processing hides, hair and wool. Endemic in numerous agricultural areas; small localized epidemics may occur. Enzootic in cattle, sheep and goats in most parts of the world.

9. *Methods of control:*

   A. Preventive measures:

   1. Animals suspected of having anthrax should be promptly isolated and treated.
   2. Post-mortem examination of animals dying of suspected anthrax should be made by a veterinarian, and with care not to contaminate soil or environment with blood or infected tissues. Carcasses should be disposed of by incineration or deep burial with quick lime.

3. Inoculation of animals with an approved vaccine when indicated.

4. Control of effluents and trade wastes of rendering plants that may handle infected animals and of factories that manufacture products using potentially contaminated hair, wool or hides.

5. Education of employees handling potentially contaminated vehicles in personal cleanliness and care of skin abrasions. Prompt medical care of all suspicious skin lesions to exclude anthrax.

6. Dust control and proper ventilation in hazardous industries.

7. Thorough washing, disinfection or sterilization, when possible, of hair, wool or hides and bone meal or other feed of animal origin, prior to further processing.

8. Hides of animals infected with anthrax must not be sold, nor carcasses used as food.

B. Control of the infected individual, contacts and environment:

1. Report to local health authority: Case report obligatory in most states and countries, Class 2A (p. 7). Report also to appropriate livestock sanitary or agriculture authority.

2. Isolation: Until lesions are healed.

3. Concurrent disinfection: Of discharges from lesions and articles soiled therewith. Spores require steam sterilization under pressure, or burning.

4. Terminal disinfection: Thorough cleaning.

5. Quarantine: None.

6. Immunization: None. Vaccines used for animals are not applicable to man.

7. Investigation of contacts and source of infection: Search for history of exposure to infected animal product and trace to origin for discovery of disease in sporadic or epizootic form. If traced to a manufacturing plant, inspect for adequacy of preventive measures outlined in 9A above.

8. Specific treatment: Penicillin, also tetracycline antibiotics; supplementary sulfadiazine or anti-anthrax serum may be useful in severe cases.

C. Epidemic measures: Epidemics in man are rare. Trace source of infection and eliminate it. In animals, epizootics may be controlled by vaccination and treatment, removal of animals from contaminated pastures, and sterilization of feed products of animal origin.

D. International measures: Sterilization of imported bone meal before use as animal feed. Sterilization of hair for use in shaving brushes; regulation of processing of imported hair, wool, hides to minimize the hazard to man.

ASCARIASIS

1. *Identification.*—A common chronic intestinal infection by a round worm. Symptoms are variable and often vague or absent; heavy infection may give digestive disturbances, abdominal pain, exaggerated reflexes, restlessness, and disturbed sleep. Live worms passed in the stools or vomited are frequently the first sign of infection. Ordinarily a mild infection, but complications may be serious and occasional deaths among children in tropical countries are related to this cause.

Identification of eggs in feces is the usual method of diagnosis.

2. *Etiologic agent.*—Ascaris lumbricoides, the large intestinal round worm of man. After ingestion, embryonated eggs hatch in the intestinal canal, larvae penetrate the wall, and reach the lungs by way of lymphatic and circulatory systems. Most larvae reaching the lungs pass into air passages, ascend bronchi, are swallowed and eventually reach the small intestine where they grow to maturity.

3. *Source and reservoir of infection.*—Infective eggs from human feces deposited in and about houses where facilities for sanitary disposal of human excreta are lacking or not used.

4. *Mode of transmission.*—By direct or indirect transmission of the embryonated eggs from soil or other contaminated material to the mouth; embryonation requires about a month. Salads and other foods eaten raw are vehicles. Contaminated soil may be carried long distances on feet or footwear into houses and conveyances.

5. *Incubation period.*—The worms reach maturity about 2 months after ingestion.

6. *Period of communicability.*—As long as mature fertilized female worms live in the intestine. Each worm produces about 20,000 eggs a day, permitting a high content of eggs in feces even when infection is light.

7. *Susceptibility and resistance.*—Susceptibility is general. Relative resistance may develop from repeated infections.

8. *Occurrence.*—A world-wide and common infection, but more frequent in moist tropical countries where prevalence may exceed 50% of a population. Children of preschool and early school age tend to be more frequently and more heavily infected than older children and adults. Area of major prevalence in the United States is lower Appalachian plateau, eastern Tennessee and surrounding areas.

9. *Methods of control:*

   A. Preventive measures:
      1. Provision of adequate facilities for proper disposal of feces and prevention of soil contamination in areas immediately adjacent to houses, particularly in play areas of children.
      2. In rural areas, privies should be so constructed as to obviate dissemination of ascarid eggs through overflow, drainage or similar circumstance.
      3. Education of all members of the family, particularly children, to use toilet facilities.
      4. Encouragement of satisfactory hygienic habits on the part of children, especially the practice of washing the hands before handling food, and after defecating.

B. Control of the infected individual, contacts and environment:
   1. Report to local health authority: Official report not ordinarily justifiable, Class 5 (p. 7).
   2. Isolation: None.
   3. Concurrent disinfection: Sanitary disposal of feces.
   4. Terminal disinfection: None.
   5. Quarantine: None.
   6. Immunization: None.
   7. Investigation of contacts and source of infection: Individual and environmental sources of infection should be sought, particularly in the persons and premises of the family.
   8. Specific treatment: Hexylresorcinol: the drug is mildly caustic and capsules must not be chewed.

C. Epidemic measures: Surveys for prevalence in highly endemic areas, public health education in sanitation of the environment and in personal hygiene, and provision of facilities for treatment.

D. International measures: None.

BARTONELLOSIS

1. *Identification.*—An illness occurring in two stages, an interval of weeks to months usually separating an initial acute febrile period and an eruptive period. The febrile period, or Oroya fever stage, is characterized by irregular fever, rapidly developing severe anemia, pain in bones and joints, and lymphadenopathy. The eruptive or verruga stage may merge with the febrile stage, but an intervening quiescent period is usual. The eruption is in crops and consists of papules or nodules resembling hemangiomas, sometimes with many small lesions, sometimes with a few tumor-like nodules. The fatality rate of untreated Oroya Fever ranges from 10 to 40%; the verruga stage is prolonged but with low fatality. Synonyms: Oroya Fever, Verruga Peruana.

   Laboratory diagnosis is by demonstration of the etiologic agent in stained smears of red blood cells during the acute stage, in sections of skin lesions during the eruptive stage, or by blood culture during either stage.

2. *Etiologic agent.*—Bartonella bacilliformis.

3. *Source and reservoir of infection.*—Source is sandfly; reservoir is blood of an infected individual: patient, convalescent, or carrier.

4. *Mode of transmission.*—By bite of sandflies of the genus Phlebotomus, primarily P. verrucarum. Not transmissible in nature from man to man.

5. *Incubation period.*—Usually 16 to 22 days but occasionally 3 or 4 months.

6. *Period of communicability.*—Prolonged; the infectious agent may be demonstrated by blood culture weeks before and up to several years after actual illness. Duration of infectivity of sandfly, unknown.

7. *Susceptibility and resistance.*—Susceptibility is general but the disease is milder in children than adults. Inapparent infections and the carrier state are known. An attack gives permanent immunity. The verruga stage may recur.

8. *Occurrence.*—Limited to certain altitudes in mountain valleys of Peru, Ecuador, and southwest Colombia where vector is present. No special predilection for age, race, or sex.

9. *Methods of control:*

A. Preventive measures:

1. Repeated spraying at appropriate intervals with DDT or other effective insecticide having residual action, of the walls of homes and other resting places of Phlebotomus. For best results, cover all homes in the endemic area.

2. Lacking means for residual insecticidal action, nightly disinsectization of quarters with liquid spray or aerosol insecticides.

3. Screening of sleeping and living quarters (25–30 mesh per inch). Spray screens at appropriate intervals with insecticide with residual action or nightly with repellent.

4. Avoid known endemic areas after sundown; otherwise carefully apply insect repellent to exposed parts of the body.

B. Control of the infected individual, contacts and environment:

1. Report to local health authority: In selected endemic areas; in most countries not a reportable disease, Class 3B (p. 7).

2. Isolation: None. The infected individual should be protected from bites of Phlebotomus (see 9A).

3. Concurrent disinfection: None.

4. Terminal disinfection: None.

5. Quarantine: None.

6. Immunization: None.

7. Investigation of contacts and source of infection: Identification of sandflies, particularly in localities where the infected person was exposed after sundown during preceding 3 to 8 weeks.

8. Specific treatment: Penicillin, erythromycin and streptomycin are all effective in reducing the fever. Blood transfusion is useful in the phase of acute anemia.

C. Epidemic measures: Intensification of case finding and systematic spraying of houses with DDT for residual effect.

D. International measures: None.

BLASTOMYCOSIS

A. North American Blastomycosis

1. *Identification.*—North American blastomycosis occurs in two clinical forms: (a) Cutaneous blastomycosis.—A chronic granulomatous disease characterized by a papule which spreads slowly and peripherally over a period of months and years, leaving an irregular central crusted ulcer with a granulomatous base. The lesions, most commonly on exposed parts of the body such as face, hands, wrists, feet and ankles, are characterized by raised papilliform to verrucous borders containing minute abscesses. Cutaneous blastomycosis persists for years and rarely becomes generalized. The typical budding fungus can be seen on direct microscopic examination and can

be cultured from marginal areas. (b) Systemic blastomycosis.—A chronic granulomatous infection, primarily of the lungs; begins with fever and symptoms of upper respiratory infection resembling influenza; progresses gradually with fever, loss of weight, cachexia with cough, purulent sputum and abscesses in subcutaneous tissues, bones, central nervous system and reproductive organs; highly fatal.

Direct examination of unstained smears of sputum and materials from lesions shows characteristic budding forms which can be cultured. A positive complement fixation test is diagnostic if histoplasmosis can be excluded.

2. *Etiologic agent.*—Blastomyces dermatitidis.

3. *Source and reservoir of infection.*—Source unknown; reservoir probably is soil or vegetation.

4. *Mode of transmission.*—Infectious agent presumably introduced through wounds or abrasions, or inhaled in spore-laden dust.

5. *Incubation period.*—Unknown; probably weeks or months.

6. *Period of communicability.*—Unknown; not directly transmissible in nature from man to man.

7. *Susceptibility and resistance.*—Unknown. Inapparent infections are probable but of undetermined frequency. No information on immunity; rarity of the disease and absence of laboratory infections suggest man is relatively resistant.

8. *Occurrence.*—Uncommon, occurring sporadically in central and southeastern United States and in Canada. Occurs at all ages, but two-thirds of cases are between 15 and 45. Males are infected seven times more frequently than females. Infection of dogs is reported with increasing frequency.

9. *Methods of control:*

   A. Preventive measures: None.

   B. Control of the infected individual, contacts and environment:

      1. Report to local health authority: Official report not ordinarily justifiable, Class 5 (p. 7).
      2. Isolation: None.
      3. Concurrent disinfection: Sputum, discharges and all contaminated articles.
      4. Terminal disinfection: Thorough cleaning.
      5. Quarantine: None.
      6. Immunization: None.
      7. Investigation of contacts and source of infection: Not profitable.
      8. Specific treatment: Recent evidence indicates stilbamidine and 2-hydroxystilbamidine are effective agents but treatment must be used with caution. Roentgen-ray therapy is helpful in cutaneous blastomycosis after partial desensitization with Blastomyces vaccine. Propamidine may be used topically.

   C. Epidemic measures: Not applicable, a sporadic disease.

   D. International measures: None.

B. South American Blastomycosis

1. *Identification.*—A chronic granulomatous infection with ulcerative lesions of skin around mouth and nose, and in tongue, cheeks and

tonsils. Other clinical types include lymphatic involvement of the neck, with or without oral lesions, and infection of lungs, spleen, kidneys, pancreas and other viscera. The cutaneous disease usually responds to treatment; systemic infection is highly fatal. Synonym: Paracoccidioidal Granuloma.

Microscopic examination of smears from lesions shows yeast-like cells with multiple buds.

2. *Etiologic agent.*—Blastomyces brasiliensis (Paracoccidioides brasiliensis).

3. *Source and reservoir of infection.*—Presumably wood or vegetation. Fungus recently demonstrated in apparently normal mouths, especially around teeth.

4. *Mode of transmission.*—Presumably acquired through contact with contaminated soil or vegetable materials or from auto-inoculation with fungi in normal mouth.

5. *Incubation period.*—Unknown.

6. *Period of communicability.*—Unknown; not directly transmissible in nature from man to man.

7. *Susceptibility and resistance.*—Unknown.

8. *Occurrence.*—Endemic in South America, particularly rural Brazil. Highest incidence in adults aged 20 to 30 years; males exceed females about ten times.

9. *Methods of control:*

   A. Preventive measures: None.

   B. Control of the infected individual, contacts and environment:

      1. Report to local health authority: Official report not ordinarily justifiable, Class 5 (p. 7).
      2. Isolation: None.
      3. Concurrent disinfection: Of discharges and contaminated articles.
      4. Terminal disinfection: Thorough cleaning.
      5. Quarantine: None.
      6. Immunization: None.
      7. Investigation of contacts and source of infection: Not profitable.
      8. Specific treatment: Stilbamidine and pentamidine.

   C. Epidemic measures: Not applicable.

   D. International measures: None.

BRUCELLOSIS

1. *Identification.*—A general infection with acute or insidious onset, characterized by continued, intermittent or irregular fever of variable duration, headache, weakness, profuse sweating, chills or chilliness, and generalized aching. The disease may last for several days, many months or occasionally for several years. Recovery is usual but disability is often pronounced. Fatality rate about 2% or less; higher for B. melitensis than other varieties. Clinical diagnosis is often difficult and uncertain. Synonym: Undulant Fever.

Laboratory diagnosis is by isolation of the infectious agent from blood, bone marrow or other tissue, or from discharges of the patient. The agglutination test is a valuable aid.

2. *Etiologic agent.*—Brucella melitensis; Brucella abortus; Brucella suis.

3. *Source and reservoir of infection.*—The sources of infection are tissues, blood, urine, milk, and especially placentas, vaginal discharges and aborted fetuses of infected animals. Reservoirs of infection are cattle, swine, sheep, goats and horses.

4. *Mode of transmission.*—By contact with infected animals, animal tissues or secretions, and by ingestion of milk and dairy products from infected animals. Air-borne infection may occur in laboratories.

5. *Incubation period.*—Highly variable and difficult to ascertain: onset is insidious and date of infection usually not established; usually 14 to 30 days, occasionally 3 months.

6. *Period of communicability.*—Rarely communicable from man to man; the infecting microorganism may be discharged in urine and other excretions for long periods.

7. *Susceptibility and resistance.*—Susceptibility is variable, as indicated by wide differences in severity and duration of clinical illness, lesser susceptibility of children to manifest disease, and frequency of mild and inapparent infections. Duration of acquired immunity is uncertain.

8. *Occurrence.*—World wide, especially Mediterranean countries of Europe and North and South America. Males affected more often than females because of occupational hazards. Sporadic cases and outbreaks occur among consumers of unpasteurized milk or milk products from cows and goats. More prevalent than present reports indicate because of diagnostic difficulties; in the United States fewer than 4,000 cases reported annually, with actual number estimated in excess of 10,000.

9. *Methods of control.*—Ultimate control in man rests in the elimination of the disease among domestic animals.

    A. Preventive measures:

        1. Education of farmers and workers in slaughterhouses, packing plants and butcher shops as to the nature of the disease and the danger of handling carcasses or products of infected animals.

        2. Search for infection among livestock by the agglutination reaction and elimination of infected animals from herds by segregation or slaughter. The control of infection among swine usually requires slaughter of the drove.

        3. Pasteurization of milk and dairy products from cows, sheep or goats. Boiling milk is practicable when pasteurization is not possible.

        4. Vaccination of calves.

        5. Care in handling and disposal of discharges and fetus from an aborted animal. Disinfection of areas contaminated.

        6. Meat inspection and condemning of carcasses of infected swine; not a useful procedure for cattle.

B. Control of the infected individual, contacts and environment:

1. Report to local health authority: Case report obligatory in most states and countries, Class 2B (p. 7).
2. Isolation: None.
3. Concurrent disinfection: Of body discharges.
4. Terminal disinfection: None.
5. Quarantine: None.
6. Immunization: None.
7. Investigation of contacts and source of infection: Trace infection to the common or individual source, usually infected domestic goats, swine, or cattle, or unpasteurized milk or dairy products from cows and goats.
8. Specific treatment: The tetracycline antibiotics usually produce prompt subsidence of fever and symptoms within several days. The relapse rate is high. More satisfactory results are obtained with a combination of chlortetracycline (aureomycin) and dihydrostreptomycin with or without the addition of a sulfonamide. Treatment should be continued for at least 3 weeks.

C. Epidemic measures: Search for common source of infection, usually unpasteurized milk or milk products from an infected herd. Stop distribution or provide pasteurization.

D. International measures: Control of domestic animals in international trade and transport.

CAT SCRATCH FEVER

1. *Identification.*—A benign infection marked by appearance within 3 to 5 days of a red or purple inflammatory lesion of the skin at the site of cat bite or trauma; resembles a furuncle and may become crusted or pustular. Two to 3 weeks after injury, with limits of 4 days to more than a month, one or more regional lymph nodes becomes enlarged, but usually solitary with overlying skin inflamed. Some patients have an evanescent rash. Symptoms of malaise, headache, anorexia and occasionally chills become more pronounced and temperature may rise to 38.9°–40° C (102°–104° F), persisting for days and weeks until rupture of suppurating lymph node. The process then subsides, healing is rapid and recovery usual. Instances of a fatal meningoencephalitis have been described. Some patients have neither cutaneous lesion nor suppurating lymph node. Synonym: Benign Inoculation Lymphoreticulosis.

A skin test and complement fixation with psittacosis-granuloma venereum group antigen are aids in diagnosis. Confirmation is by inoculation of monkeys with material from local lesions or discharges from suppurating lymph nodes.

2. *Etiologic agent.*—Unknown; a virus closely related to the psittacosis-lymphogranuloma venereum group has been isolated from lesions.

3. *Source and reservoir of infection.*—Probably several animals, usually with inapparent infection, of which the domestic cat is best known.

4. *Mode of transmission.*—Commonly by bite, scratch or lick of a cat, or exposure to other animals including birds, or bite of an insect. Frequent absence of such exposure suggests other modes of transmission, as through minor trauma after thorn scratch, or puncture by splinters of wood, spicules of bone or porcupine quill.

5. *Incubation period.*—Several days; 2 to 8 days in instances of definite trauma.

6. *Period of communicability.*—Unknown for reservoir host or for man; in man presumably for duration of open lesions; not known to be communicable from man to man.

7. *Susceptibility and resistance.*—Unknown.

8. *Occurrence.*—Apparently universal; reported from nearly every country in Europe, from South Africa, the United States and Canada, and several countries in South America. Commonly sporadic with occasional family or community outbreaks. Seasonal variation not determined; sex distribution equal; approximately one-third of patients are aged less than 10 years; more than one-half are under 20 years.

9. *Methods of control:*

   A. Preventive measures:

      1. A disease first recognized in 1950. No definite preventive measures, other than avoidance of cats.

   B. Control of the infected individual, contacts and environment:

      1. Report to local health authority: Official report not ordinarily justifiable, Class 5 (p. 7).
      2. Isolation: None.
      3. Concurrent disinfection: Of discharges from cutaneous lesions or lymph nodes.
      4. Terminal disinfection: None.
      5. Quarantine: None.
      6. Immunization: None.
      7. Investigation of contacts and source of infection: Examination of family contacts for common exposure and search for cats as possible reservoirs.
      8. Specific treatment: None; chloramphenicol and tetracycline antibiotics are stated to shorten the course.

   C. Epidemic measures: None.

   D. International measures: None.

CHANCROID

1. *Identification.*—An acute, localized, self-limiting autoinoculable infectious disease characterized clinically by necrotizing ulcerations at the site of inoculation. Genital lesions frequently are accompanied by painful inflammatory swelling and suppuration of regional lymph nodes. Extragenital lesions of umbilicus, tongue, lip, breast, chin and bulbar conjunctiva are on record. Synonyms: Ulcus Molle, Chancre Mou, Soft Chancre and Soft Sore.

Microscopic examination of stained exudate from edges of lesion, bacteriologic culture of pus from buboes, intradermal skin test, autoinoculation and biopsy are diagnostic aids.

2. *Etiologic agent.*—Hemophilus ducreyi, Ducrey bacillus.

3. *Source and reservoir of infection.*—Patients with discharges from open lesions and pus from buboes; suggestive evidence that women are occasionally carriers.

4. *Mode of transmission.*—Predominantly venereal except for rare instances of professionally acquired lesions on hands of doctors and nurses; also accidental inoculation of children. Indirect transmission is rare. Prostitution, indiscriminate sexual promiscuity and uncleanliness are important factors favoring transmission.

5. *Incubation period.*—3 to 5 days, occasionally longer; if abrasions of mucous membrane are present, as short as 24 hours.

6. *Period of communicability.*—As long as the etiologic agent persists in the original lesion or discharging regional lymph nodes; usually parallels healing and in most instances a matter of weeks.

7. *Susceptibility and resistance.*—Susceptibility is general; no evidence of natural or acquired immunity.

8. *Occurrence.*—No particular differences in incidence according to age, race or sex except as determined by sexual habits. Geographically widespread and in some areas a relatively frequent disease. Incidence in military forces is sometimes higher than for syphilis.

9. *Methods of control:*

    A. Preventive measures:

        1. Except for specific reference to chancroid as such, and those measures specific for syphilis, the preventive measures are those of syphilis (see 9A, p. 178).

    B. Control of the infected individual, contacts and environment:

        1. Report to local health authority: Case report obligatory in many states and countries, Class 2B (p. 7).

        2. Isolation: None; avoid sexual contact until lesions are healed.

        3. Concurrent disinfection: None; ordinary personal cleanliness.

        4. Terminal disinfection: None.

        5. Quarantine: None.

        6. Immunization: None.

        7. Investigation of contacts and source of infection: Search for sexual contacts of the period 2 weeks before lesions appeared and after signs and symptoms became evident.

        8. Specific treatment: Sulfonamides (sulfanilamide, sulfathiazole or sulfadiazine); tetracycline antibiotics (aureomycin) and chloramphenicol only in case of sulfonamide resistance because of the potentiality of masking syphilis.

    C. Epidemic measures: Non-declining levels of occurrence or any increase in incidence are indication for increased vigilance and more rigid application of measures outlined in 9A and 9B.

    D. International measures: (See Syphilis 9D, p. 179).

CHICKENPOX

1. *Identification.*—An acute infectious disease of sudden onset with slight fever, mild constitutional symptoms and an eruption which is maculopapular for a few hours, vesicular for 3 to 4 days, and leaves a granular scab. Lesions tend to be more abundant on covered than on exposed parts of the body; may appear on scalp, and mucous membrane of upper respiratory tract; commonly occur in successive crops with several stages of maturity present at the same time; may be so few as to escape observation. Essentially nonfatal; such deaths as occur are almost invariably the result of septic complications or encephalitis. Synonym: Varicella.

    Laboratory tests for identification of variola virus are sometimes necessary to distinguish chickenpox from smallpox.

2. *Etiologic agent.*—The virus of chickenpox; whether the agent is an independent virus or identical with that of herpes zoster remains controversial.

3. *Source and reservoir of infection.*—Secretions of the respiratory tract of infected persons; lesions of the skin are of little consequence and scabs of themselves are not infective.

4. *Mode of transmission.*—From person to person by direct contact or droplet spread; indirectly through articles freshly soiled by discharges from the skin and mucous membranes of infected persons. One of the most readily communicable of diseases, especially in the early stages of the eruption.

5. *Incubation period.*—2 to 3 weeks; commonly 13 to 17 days.

6. *Period of communicability.*—Probably not more than one day before nor more than 6 days after the appearance of the first crop of vesicles.

7. *Susceptibility and resistance.*—Susceptibility is universal among those not previously attacked; ordinarily a more severe disease of adults than of children. An attack confers long immunity; second attacks are rare.

8. *Occurrence.*—Nearly universal. In metropolitan communities probably 70 percent of persons have had the disease by 15 years of age. Not uncommon in early infancy. Winter is the season of greatest prevalence in temperate zones.

9. *Methods of control:*

    A. Preventive measures:
    1. The chief public health importance of this disease is that cases thought to be chickenpox in persons over 15 years, or of any age during an epidemic of smallpox, should be viewed with suspicion and investigated to eliminate possibility of smallpox.

    B. Control of the infected individual, contacts and environment:
    1. Report to local health authority: Official report is not ordinarily justifiable, Class 5 (p. 7). Case report of chickenpox in adults (Class 3B) may be required where smallpox is infrequent.
    2. Isolation: Exclusion from school for the period of communicability, and avoidance of contact with non-immune persons.

34

    3. Concurrent disinfection: Articles soiled by discharges from the nose and throat and from lesions.

    4. Terminal disinfection: None.

    5. Quarantine: None.

    6. Immunization: None.

    7. Investigation of contacts and source of infection: Of no importance.

    8. Specific treatment: None.

C. Epidemic measures: No procedures in common use can be relied upon as a means of effective control of the disease or of epidemics.

D. International measures: None.

CHOLERA

1. *Identification.*—A serious acute intestinal infection characterized by sudden onset, vomiting, profuse watery diarrhea, rapid dehydration and collapse. Severity differs greatly from place to place and within epidemics; mild cases show only diarrhea. Death may occur within 24 hours. Epidemics tend to be explosive and fatality varies from 10 to 80%.

    Cholera vibrios can be cultivated from feces; if abundant, can be recognized on direct smear.

2. *Etiologic agent.*—Vibrio cholerae, cholera vibrio.

3. *Source and reservoir of infection.*—Feces and vomitus of patients, feces of persons incubating the disease and of convalescents.

4. *Mode of transmission.*—Fecal contamination of water; of foods by soiled hands, utensils, or flies. Carriers do not play a significant role in spread of the infection.

5. *Incubation period.*—From a few hours to 5 days, usually 3 days.

6. *Period of communicability.*—While cholera vibrios are present in feces, usually 7 to 14 days after onset.

7. *Susceptibility and resistance.*—Susceptibility is general, although variable. Frank clinical attack confers a temporary immunity which may afford some protection for several years. Immunity artificially induced by vaccines is of variable degree and uncertain duration.

8. *Occurrence.*—Endemic in parts of India and certain adjacent areas of Southeast Asia. From these centers, spreads along lines of communication, from time to time reaching remote countries and causing widespread epidemics. Absent from Europe and Western Hemisphere for many years although has invaded repeatedly.

9. *Methods of control:*

A. Preventive measures:

    1. Sanitary disposal of human feces.

    2. Protection and purification of public water supplies and construction of safe private supplies.

    3. Boiling of milk or pasteurization of milk and dairy products.

4. Sanitary supervision of processing, preparation, and serving of foods, especially those that are moist and eaten raw; special attention to provision and use of hand-washing facilities.

5. Fly control, control of fly breeding and screening to protect foods against fly contamination.

6. Education of public in habits of personal cleanliness, especially washing hands before eating and after defecation.

7. Active immunization with cholera vaccine of persons subject to unusual risk.

B. Control of the infected individual, contacts and environment:

1. Report to local health authority: Case report universally required by international regulation, Class 1 (p. 6).

2. Isolation: Of patient in hospital or screened room during communicable period.

3. Concurrent disinfection: Prompt and thorough disinfection of feces and vomitus, and of articles used by patient. Practice by attendants of scrupulous cleanliness; disinfection of hands each time after handling or touching articles contaminated by feces.

4. Terminal disinfection: Thorough cleaning.

5. Quarantine: Surveillance of contacts for 5 days from last exposure and longer if feces contain cholera vibrio.

6. Immunization: No passive immunization. Inoculation of contacts with cholera vaccine can be expected to do no more than protect against subsequent or continued exposure. (See C3 infra.)

7. Investigation of contacts and source of infection: Search for unreported cases and carriers. Investigate possible infection from polluted drinking water or from contaminated uncooked foods.

8. Specific treatment: None. Replacement of fluid and electrolyte and other measures for shock are paramount.

C. Epidemic measures:

1. Boiling of water used for drinking, toilet purposes, or washing dishes or food containers, unless water supply is adequately treated as by chlorination.

2. Inspection service for early detection of infected persons; provision of temporary emergency facilities for isolation of patients and suspects; identification and isolation of carriers desirable but usually impracticable; detention in suitable camps for 5 days, of those desirous of leaving for another locality.

3. Immediate administration of cholera vaccine to exposed population groups, despite its uncertain value.

4. Careful supervision of food and drink. After cooking or boiling should be protected against contamination, as by flies and human handling.

5. Control of flies, by limiting fly breeding, by use of appropriate insecticides and by screening kitchens and eating places.

D. International measures:

1. Telegraphic notification of WHO and of adjacent countries, by governments, of the existence of an epidemic of cholera.

2. Measures applicable to ships, aircraft and land transport arriving from cholera areas are specified in International Sanitary Regulations (WHO Techn. Rept. Ser. No. 41, Geneva, 1951).

3. International travellers: Most countries within endemic areas, particularly Southeast Asia, require recent inoculation with cholera vaccine for entry; many other countries have the same requirement for travellers returning from those countries. International cholera immunization certificate is valid from 6 days until 6 months after the first injection of vaccine, or in the event of revaccination within such period of 6 months as of that date and for 6 months thereafter.

CHROMOBLASTOMYCOSIS

1. *Identification.*—A chronic, spreading but strictly localized infection of the skin and subcutaneous tissues, usually of a lower extremity, occasionally upper. Progression of the lesion is slow, over a period of years, with eventual large verrucous or even cauliflower-like masses, but of itself rarely a cause of death. Synonyms: Chromomycosis, Dermatitis Verrucosa.

   Microscopic examination of scrapings from lesions reveals characteristic brown fungus spores which can be cultured.

2. *Etiologic agent.*—Phialophora verrucosa and several species of Hormodendrum (Fonsecaea).

3. *Source and reservoir of infection.*—Presumably wood or vegetation.

4. *Mode of transmission.*—Infection presumably acquired from traumatic contact with contaminated wood or other materials.

5. *Incubation period.*—Unknown; probably weeks or months.

6. *Period of communicability.*—Unknown; not transmissible from man to man.

7. *Susceptibility and resistance.*—Unknown, but rarity of disease and absence of laboratory infections suggest man is relatively resistant.

8. *Occurrence.*—Sporadic cases have been reported from widely scattered areas in the United States, Europe and Africa, with the highest incidence in South America and the West Indies; primarily a disease of rural tropical regions. The infection occurs most commonly between ages 30 and 50. Females are rarely infected.

9. *Methods of control:*

   A. Preventive measures: None.

   B. Control of the infected individual, contacts and environment:

   1. Report to local health authority: Official report not ordinarily justifiable, Class 5 (p. 7).

   2. Isolation: None.

3. Concurrent disinfection: Of discharges from lesions and articles soiled therewith.

4. Terminal disinfection: None.

5. Quarantine: None.

6. Immunization: None.

7. Investigation of contacts and source of infection: Not profitable.

8. Specific treatment: None; iodides, copper sulfate and sulphur should be tried. Stilbamidine or 2-hydroxystilbamidine may be used with care systemically, and propamidine locally.

C. Epidemic measures: Not applicable, a sporadic disease.

D. International measures: None.

CLONORCHIASIS

1. *Identification.*—An infection of the bile ducts with Clonorchis sinensis, the Asiatic liver fluke of man. Clinical effects may be slight or absent in light infection. Symptoms result from local irritation of bile ducts by flukes, from systemic toxemia and possibly from secondary bacterial invaders. Loss of appetite, diarrhea and sensations of abdominal pressure are common first symptoms. Bile duct obstruction, rarely producing jaundice, may be followed by cirrhosis, enlargement and tenderness of the liver, and progressive ascites and edema. Eosinophilia is frequent, 5 to 40%. A long continued disease, sometimes 20 years or more, but uncommonly either a direct or contributing cause of death. Synonym: Chinese Liver Fluke Disease.

Direct diagnosis depends on finding the characteristic fluke eggs in feces or by duodenal drainage. Differentiation is required from eggs of heterophyid and opisthorchid flukes, producing disease in cats and dogs but also heterophydiasis and opisthorchiasis in man in Southeast Asia, Egypt, Russia and other countries.

2. *Etiologic agent.*—Clonorchis sinensis.

3. *Source and reservoir of infection.*—Fresh water fish eaten raw (fresh, dried, salted or pickled) or partly cooked. Man, cat, dog, hog and other animals are reservoir hosts of adult flukes.

4. *Mode of transmission.*—Eggs deposited in the bile passages are evacuated in feces. Eggs in feces contain a fully developed miracidium; if ingested by a susceptible snail (Buliminae of the family Amnicolidae), hatches in its intestine and penetrates vascular spaces. Cercariae develop and emerge into water; on contact with second intermediate host, fresh-water fishes (Cyprinidae) of which 40 or more species are appropriate, cercariae penetrate the host and encyst, usually in muscle, occasionally on underside of scales. Man or other definitive host is infected by eating fish; during digestion larvae are set free from cysts, and migrate via the common bile duct to biliary capillaries. The complete life cycle, from man to man, requires at least 3 months.

5. *Incubation period.*—Undetermined; flukes reach egg-producing maturity by 16th to 25th day after encysted larvae are ingested.

6. *Period of communicability.*—As long as viable eggs are passed in feces; may be 15 to 20 years.

7. *Susceptibility and resistance.*—Susceptibility is general. No resistance develops with age; in endemic areas, highest incidence at 55 to 60 years.

8. *Occurrence.*—Highly endemic in southeast China, present in all parts except northwest; Japan, widespread; Formosa; south Korea; and French Indo-China, principally Red River Delta. Imported cases in immigrants in other parts of the world. Native Hawaiians contract disease from fish imported from China or Japan. An epidemic of some 5,000 cases occurred among European refugees in Shanghai in 1946.

9. *Methods of control:*

   A. Preventive measures:

      1. In endemic areas, education of the public regarding life cycle of parasite.
      2. Thorough cooking of all fresh-water fish.
      3. Treatment or storage of nightsoil before use as fertilizer in fish ponds; 1 part of 0.7% solution of ammonium sulphate to 10 parts of feces will kill eggs in 30 minutes.

   B. Control of the infected individual, contacts and environment:

      1. Report to local health authority: In selected endemic areas; in most countries not a reportable disease, Class 3C (p. 7).
      2. Isolation: None.
      3. Concurrent disinfection: Sanitary disposal of feces.
      4. Terminal disinfection: None.
      5. Quarantine: None.
      6. Immunization: None.
      7. Investigation of contacts and source of infection: Of the individual case, unprofitable. A community problem (see 9C).
      8. Specific treatment: None; gentian violet medicinal is clonorchicidal and appears to be of some value.

   C. Epidemic measures: Locate source of infected fish parasitized through use of nightsoil as fertilizer in fish ponds, or through fecal contamination of streams. Shipments of dried or pickled fish are the likely source in non-endemic areas.

   D. International measures: None.

COCCIDIOIDOMYCOSIS

1. *Identification.*—

   A. Primary infection: May be entirely asymptomatic or resemble an acute febrile influenzal illness, with fever, chills, cough, and pleural pain. About one-fifth of clinically recognized cases (an estimated 5% of all primary infections) develop erythema nodosum (Valley Fever); or more rarely erythema multiforme, a complication most frequent in white females and rarest in Negro males. Primary infection may (1) heal completely without detectable residuals, (2) leave radiographic fibrosis or calcification of pulmonary lesions, (3) leave a persistent thin-walled cavity, or (4) and most rarely, progress to the disseminated form of the disease, comparable to progressive primary tuberculosis.

The fungus may be found in sputum by direct examination or by culture. Reaction to skin test with coccidioidin appears within two days to three weeks after onset; precipitin and complement fixation tests are usually positive at an early date.

B. Coccidioidal granuloma: A progressive, highly fatal granulomatous disease characterized by lung lesions and single or multiple abscesses throughout the body, especially in subcutaneous tissues, skin, bone, peritoneum, testes, thyroid and central nervous system. Coccidioidal meningitis resembles tuberculous meningitis.

The fungus can be demonstrated in sputum and in materials from lesions by microscopic examination or by culture.

A granulomatous disease, sometimes referred to as paracoccidioidal granuloma, has no relationship to coccidioidomycosis (see South American Blastomycosis, p. 28).

2. *Etiologic agent.*—Coccidioides immitis.

3. *Source and reservoir of infection.*—Source is soil contaminated with spores of the fungus. Reservoir of infection is unknown.

4. *Mode of transmission.*—Inhalation of spores in dust and dry vegetation, and in laboratories inhalation of spores from cultures. Infection through open wounds is a possible but infrequent route. Not directly transmissible in nature from man to man.

5. *Incubation period.*—Ten days to three weeks in primary infection. Coccidioidal granuloma develops insidiously, not necessarily preceded by symptoms of primary pulmonary infection.

6. *Period of communicability.*—Contamination of environment as long as open lesions remain.

7. *Susceptibility and resistance.*—Susceptibility to primary infection is general; high incidence of positive coccidioidin reactors in endemic areas; recovery apparently is followed by solid immunity.

8. *Occurrence.*—Primary infections are extremely common in scattered, highly endemic arid areas; in United States from California to West Texas, and in South America several areas having similar climate and terrain. Affects all ages, both sexes, and all races. Infection most frequent in summer, especially after wind and dust storms. Coccidioidal granuloma has the geographic distribution of Valley Fever. More than half of cases occur between 15 and 35 years of age; males are infected five times as frequently as females; and dark-skinned individuals ten times more than others.

9. *Methods of control:*

A. Preventive measures:

1. In endemic areas, planting of grass, oiling and other dust-control measures. Individuals from non-endemic areas should not be recruited to dusty occupations such as road-building.

B. Control of the infected individual, contacts and environment:

1. Report to local health authority: Case report of clinically recognized coccidioidal infection in selected endemic areas (USA); in many countries not a reportable disease, Class 3B (p. 7).

2. Isolation: None.

3. Concurrent disinfection: Of discharges and soiled articles.
4. Terminal disinfection: Thorough cleaning.
5. Quarantine: None.
6. Immunization: None.
7. Investigation of contacts and source of infection: Not profitable.
8. Specific treatment: None.

C. Epidemic measures: Epidemics occur only when groups of susceptibles are infected by air-borne spores. Dust control measures should be instituted where practicable.

D. International measures: None.

COLORADO TICK FEVER, VIRAL

1. *Identification.*—An acute febrile, erythematous disease without macular rash, usually with brief remission followed by a second bout of fever, each of two or three days duration; no reported deaths.

   Specific serological tests using mouse adapted virus are used in laboratory confirmation of diagnosis.

   Clinical course, symptomatology and leucocyte response are almost identical with Dengue; to be differentiated from Rocky Mountain Spotted Fever.

2. *Etiologic agent.*—The virus of Colorado tick fever.

3. *Source and reservoir of infection.*—Source of infection is vector ticks, usually Dermacentor andersoni. Reservoir is the blood of infected persons; also ticks because of transovarian passage of the agent. An animal reservoir other than man probably exists but has not been demonstrated.

4. *Mode of transmission.*—Ticks presumably acquire infection through feeding on infected animals during period of viremia and after suitable extrinsic incubation transmit to man by feeding. Transovarian transmission by infected ticks has been demonstrated.

5. *Incubation period.*—Usually 4 to 5 days.

6. *Period of communicability.*—Not directly communicable in nature from man to man. Virus is present in man during febrile course, from 1 to 10 days after onset.

7. *Susceptibility and resistance.*—Susceptibility apparently universal. Second attacks are unknown; experimental reinfection unsuccessful.

8. *Occurrence.*—Known area of occurrence limited to United States; Oregon, Utah, Idaho, Wyoming, Montana and Colorado; a similar virus reported from Dermacentor variabilis Long Island, New York, but disease in man not recognized. Predominantly a disease of adults; seasonal incidence corresponds to greatest tick activity; sporadic and endemic distribution; an uncommon disease even in affected areas.

9. *Methods of control:*

   A. Preventive measures:
      1. Control of ticks; see Rocky Mountain Spotted Fever, 9 A1 and 2 (pp. 156–7).
      2. No available vaccine.

B. Control of the infected individual, contacts and environment:
1. Report to local health authority: In endemic areas (USA); in most states and countries not a reportable disease, Class 3B (p. 7).
2. Isolation: None.
3. Concurrent disinfection: None; all ticks on patient should be destroyed.
4. Terminal disinfection: None.
5. Quarantine: None.
6. Immunization: None.
7. Investigation of contacts and source of infection: Identification of ticks and tick infested areas.
8. Specific treatment: None.

C. Epidemic measures: Not applicable.

D. International measures: None.

COMMON COLD

1. *Identification.*—An acute catarrhal infection of the upper respiratory tract characterized by coryza, lacrimation, irritated nasopharynx, chilliness and malaise lasting 2 to 7 days. Probably never fatal; importance rests in days of disability and in predisposing to more serious respiratory tract infections. Fever is uncommon, particularly in infants and adults. Complications of catarrhal sinusitis, otitis media, laryngitis, tracheitis or bronchitis are frequent.

No confirmatory laboratory tests; leucocyte count and distribution are normal.

The common cold, as here described, is to be differentiated from other minor respiratory illnesses which in general are more severe, with fever and constitutional symptoms, and an incubation period in experimentally infected volunteers of from 4 to 6 days or longer. Examples are Acute Respiratory Disease (ARD), Catarrhal Fever, and Non-bacterial Exudative Tonsillitis and Pharyngitis.

2. *Etiologic agent.*—The infection has been transmitted experimentally to chimpanzees and man by a filter-passing agent, presumably a virus. Cultivation and characterization not achieved; more than one type is probable but undetermined. Role of bacteria in the usual case is uncertain; pyogenic bacteria of respiratory tract (pneumococci, streptococci, H. influenzae) may cause suppurative complications.

3. *Source and reservoir of infection.*—Discharges from nose and mouth of patients.

4. *Mode of transmission.*—Usual transmission is by direct contact or by droplet spread; indirectly by handkerchiefs, eating utensils or other articles freshly soiled by discharges of the infected person.

5. *Incubation period.*—Between 12 and 72 hours, usually 24 hours.

6. *Period of communicability.*—Nasal washings taken 24 hours before onset and for 5 days after onset produce symptoms experimentally in man.

7. *Susceptibility and resistance.*—Susceptibility is universal. Inapparent and abortive attacks occur; frequency undetermined. Epidemiological evidence suggests limited and transient immunity; no im-

munity demonstrated in volunteers re-inoculated after 3 weeks. No artificial immunization.

8. *Occurrence.*—World-wide distribution; endemic and epidemic. In temperate zones, incidence rises during winter months. Most persons, except in small isolated communities, have 1 to 6 colds yearly. Incidence highest in children under 5 years; gradual decline with increasing age.

9. *Methods of control:*

A. Preventive measures:

1. Education in the niceties of personal hygiene as in covering the mouth when coughing and sneezing and disposal of nose and mouth secretions.

B. Control of the infected individual, contacts and environment:

1. Report to local health authority: Official report not ordinarily justifiable, Class 5 (p. 7).

2. Isolation: On first recognition of a common cold the infected person should avoid direct and indirect exposure of others, particularly little children, feeble or aged persons, or persons suffering from other illness. Such modified isolation as can be accomplished by rest in bed during the acute stage is advised.

3. Concurrent disinfection: Of eating and drinking utensils; disposal of nose and mouth discharges, preferably by collecting on soft paper and burning.

4. Terminal disinfection: Airing and sunning of room and bedding.

5. Quarantine: None.

6. Immunization: None.

7. Investigation of contacts and source of infection: Unprofitable.

8. Specific treatment: None. Indiscriminate use of antibiotics for uncomplicated colds or mild sore throat is to be discouraged. These valuable therapeutic agents should be reserved for complications such as pneumonia, tracheobronchitis, otitis, and sinusitis.

C. Epidemic measures: Effective measures for the control of epidemics are not known. Isolation precautions may be helpful in institutions but procedures such as ultraviolet irradiation, aerosols and dust control have not been effective.

D. International measures: None.

CONJUNCTIVITIS, ACUTE BACTERIAL

1. *Identification.*—The disease begins with lacrimation, irritation, and vascular injection of the palpebral and bulbar conjunctivae of one or both eyes, followed by edema of the lids, photophobia, pain and a mucopurulent exudate; in severe cases, ecchymoses of the bulbar conjunctiva and transient phlyctenules on the cornea. A non-fatal disease with usual clinical course of 2 to 3 weeks; many patients have no more than vascular injection of the conjunctivae and slight exudate for a few days. Synonyms: Sore Eyes, Pink Eye.

Confirmation by bacteriologic culture, or microscopic examination of smears of exudate.

Other forms of acute conjunctivitis are to be differentiated: acute conjunctivitis of the newborn to include gonorrheal ophthalmia, ophthalmia neonatorum and babies' sore eyes of the first 21 days of life (p. 79), trachoma (p. 186), keratoconjunctivitis (p. 92) and inclusion blenorrhea.

2. *Etiologic agent.*—Haemophilus aegyptius (Koch-Weeks bacillus) appears to be the most important; Haemophilus influenzae, Moraxella lacunatus, staphylococci, streptococci, pneumococci and C. diphtheriae may produce the disease.

3. *Source and reservoir of infection.*—Discharges from the conjunctiva or upper respiratory tract of infected persons, possibly including chronic carriers.

4. *Mode of transmission.*—Contact with infected individuals through contaminated fingers, clothing or other fomites. In some areas may be mechanically transmitted by eye-gnats or flies, but importance as a vector undetermined and probably differs from area to area.

5. *Incubation period.*—Usually 24 to 72 hours.

6. *Period of communicability.*—During the course of active infection.

7. *Susceptibility and resistance.*—Children under 5 are most often affected and incidence decreases with age. The debilitated and aged are particularly susceptible to staphylococcal infections. Immunity after attack is low-grade and variable, according to the infectious agent involved.

8. *Occurrence.*—Widespread throughout the world, particularly in warmer climates; frequently epidemic. In the United States, infection with H. aegyptius is largely confined to rural areas of southernmost states, Georgia to California, primarily during summer and early autumn months; in those areas an important cause of absenteeism from school. Infection with other organisms occurs throughout the United States, often associated with acute respiratory infection during cold seasons.

9. *Methods of control:*

A. Preventive measures:

1. Personal cleanliness, hygienic care, and treatment of affected eyes.

B. Control of the infected individual, contacts, and environment:

1. Report to local health authority: Obligatory report of epidemics; no case report, Class 4 (p. 7).

2. Isolation: Children should not attend school during the acute stage.

3. Concurrent disinfection: Of discharges and soiled articles.

4. Terminal disinfection: Thorough cleaning.

5. Quarantine: None.

6. Immunization: None.

7. Investigation of contacts and source of infection: Usually not profitable.

8. Specific treatment: Local application of a tetracycline antibiotic (aureomycin, terramycin), streptomycin or penicillin, the latter primarily for the less common streptococcal and pneumococcal infections.

C. Epidemic measures:
  1. Adequate and intensive treatment of patients and their associates.
  2. In areas where insects are suspected of mechanically transmitting infection, measures to prevent access of eye-gnats or flies to eyes of sick and well persons.
  3. Insect control, depending on the suspected vector.

D. International measures: None.

CRYPTOCOCCOSIS

1. *Identification.*—The most frequently recognized form of the infection in the United States is a chronic, almost invariably fatal meningitis (Torula meningitis). The fungus also produces acne-like skin lesions, subcutaneous tumor-like masses, pulmonary lesions and occasionally a generalized infection involving diverse organs. Synonyms: Torulosis, European Blastomycosis.

    Cryptococcus meningitis is recognized by careful microscopic examination of spinal fluid. The fungus should be cultured and pathogenicity determined.

2. *Etiologic agent.*—Cryptococcus neoformans (Torula histolytica).

3. *Source and reservoir of infection.*—Source is skin and gastro-intestinal tract of normal persons. Reservoir unknown; present in cattle, dogs and cats, also soil and fruit.

4. *Mode of transmission.*—Method of transmission from potential reservoirs is unknown. Not directly transmissible in nature from man to man.

5. *Incubation period.*—Unknown. Roentgenographic examination has demonstrated inapparent pulmonary infection prior to meningitis.

6. *Period of communicability.*—Unknown.

7. *Susceptibility and resistance.*—Unknown. The sporadic occurrence of meningitis and frequent finding of the fungus in normal persons suggests an appreciable resistance.

8. *Occurrence.*—Occasional sporadic cases occur in all parts of the world. All races susceptible; males infected twice as frequently as females; all ages affected but highest incidence is between 20 and 40 years.

9. *Methods of control:*

    A. Preventive measures: None.

    B. Control of the infected individual, contacts and environment:
      1. Report to local health authority: Official report ordinarily not justifiable, Class 5 (p. 7).
      2. Isolation: None.
      3. Concurrent disinfection: None.
      4. Terminal disinfection: None.
      5. Quarantine: None.
      6. Immunization: None.
      7. Investigation of source of infection: Not profitable.
      8. Specific treatment: None; actidione has been used with equivocal results.

    C. Epidemic measures: Not applicable, a sporadic disease.

    D. International measures: None.

DENGUE

1. *Identification.*—An acute febrile infection of sharp onset, occasionally with two paroxysms of short duration; fever of about five days and rarely more than seven, intense headache, joint and muscle pains, and eruption. Eruption usually appears 3 to 4 days after onset of fever, either maculopapular or scarlatiniform; petechiae may appear on feet, legs, axillae, or palate on last day of fever or shortly thereafter. Leucopenia is usual with an absolute decrease of segmented neutrophiles and a marked increase of nonsegmented forms. Epidemics are explosive and fatality is exceedingly low. Synonym: Breakbone Fever.

   Laboratory tests contributing to identification include hemagglutination, complement fixation, or neutralization techniques, using specific type of virus.

2. *Etiologic agent.*—The viruses of dengue fever; at least two immunologically distinct types have been identified.

3. *Source and reservoir of infection.*—The immediate source of infection is an infected vector mosquito. The infected person is one reservoir; the existence of an added animal reservoir is suspected but not demonstrated.

4. *Mode of transmission.*—By the bite of mosquitoes, Aëdes aegypti, Aëdes albopictus, or one of the Aëdes scutellaris complex, infected by biting a patient.

5. *Incubation period.*—Three to 15 days, commonly 5 or 6 days.

6. *Period of communicability.*—Not directly communicable in nature from man to man. Patients are infective for mosquitoes from the day before onset to the 5th day of disease. The mosquito becomes infective from 8 to 11 days after the blood meal and remains so for life.

7. *Susceptibility and resistance.*—Susceptibility is apparently universal. Homologous immunity to either type of virus is of long duration; heterologous immunity, though present, is brief and may permit mild febrile illness without rash.

8. *Occurrence.*—Endemic areas are limited to parts of the world where mosquito vectors survive in large numbers throughout the year; also may depend on continued immigration of susceptibles such as occurs during war and on distant military posts. Islands of the Southwest Pacific, Indo-China, Indonesia, India, and northern Australia are areas commonly involved. Epidemics can occur wherever the vectors are present.

9. *Methods of control:*

   A. Preventive measures:

      1. Measures directed toward elimination of vector mosquitoes, and where practicable their breeding places.

      2. Screening of rooms.

      3. Use of mosquito repellents.

   B. Control of the infected individual, contacts and environment:

      1. Report to local health authority: Obligatory report of epidemics; no case report, Class 4 (p. 7).

46

2. Isolation: Patient should be kept in screened room for 5 days after onset, or in quarters treated with insecticide with residual effect, such as DDT.

3. Concurrent disinfection: None.

4. Terminal disinfection: None.

5. Quarantine: None.

6. Immunization: None.

7. Investigation of contacts and source of infection: Place of residence of patient during fortnight previous to onset. Search for unreported or undiagnosed cases. Determine density of Aëdes mosquitoes in vicinity and search for breeding places.

8. Specific treatment: None.

C. Epidemic measures:

1. Community survey for breeding places of vector mosquitoes, and their elimination.

2. Search for and destruction of Aëdes mosquitoes in places of human habitation.

3. Use of mosquito repellents by persons exposed through occupation or necessity to bites of vector mosquitoes.

D. International measures:

1. Enforcement of provisions of international agreements designed to prevent mosquito transfer by public conveyances (ships, airplanes, land transport) from areas of prevalence to areas free of the disease.

DIARRHEA OF THE NEWBORN, EPIDEMIC

A variety of diseases of children aged less than 2 years, having diarrhea and usually fever as the common clinical manifestation is grouped under the general term of infantile enteritis. Two broad classes are recognized. The larger and generally more serious group includes specific infections that result in primary infectious enteritis. Some are due to known pathogenic agents such as Salmonella (p. 72) and Shigella (p. 58); some are associated with serologically recognizable types of Escherichia coli or a number of other common bacteria; and others may be caused by filtrable viruses. The second class includes various forms of secondary enteritis associated with parenteral infection. The several kinds of primary enteritis cannot be distinguished accurately by clinical methods. A number are seen principally among older infants; any one may attack the newborn.

A form of acute enteritis of the newborn has characteristics sufficiently distinctive to be recognized individually; as an epidemiologic entity by reason of its practical limitation to outbreaks among infants housed in hospital nurseries, and as a clinical entity by manifestations which set it apart from the usual infantile diarrhea. It is probably not an etiologic entity. This is the condition now presented as epidemic diarrhea of the newborn.

1. *Identification.*—An acute communicable disease characterized by severe diarrhea with watery feces containing little or no mucus and no blood, by dehydration, and commonly acidosis. Signs other than of enteric infection are lacking in uncomplicated cases; the tem-

perature is normal or only slightly elevated except with severe dehydration or with pneumonia or other complication. The disorder spreads rapidly from infant to infant in a nursery for the newborn and ordinarily has a high case fatality, which varies from 0 to 40%.

Stool culture serves to identify specific infection with known pathogenic bacteria but is of no help in viral infections. Postmortem examination shows remarkably few changes and none pathognomonic of the disorder.

2. *Etiologic agent.*—Still doubtful, but probably more than one infectious agent is responsible. Some outbreaks have been attributed to a filtrable virus; others are associated with the presence in the intestine of serologically recognizable types of E. coli, 0–111, 0–55 and others.

3. *Source and Reservoir of infection.*—Unknown; presumably feces of infected persons. The specific types of E. coli appear to be present only among patients and close contacts. Nurses, physicians, and other adults sometimes serve as healthy carriers.

4. *Mode of transmission.*—Direct or indirect person to person transfer. Faults in aseptic nursing technic are a principal factor in many outbreaks, as with milk formulas and rubber nipples. In epidemics associated with specific types of E. coli, the whole of the patient's environment is contaminated and the organism can be demonstrated on bed clothing and in dust of the ward.

5. *Incubation period.*—Unknown; estimates are from 2 to 21 days, most frequently 6 to 7 days.

6. *Period of communicability.*—Readily communicable among newborn infants as long as symptoms are present or a carrier state persists.

7. *Susceptibility and resistance.*—Restricted in general to infants under one month of age, most frequently those 8 to 9 days old. Premature infants are more susceptible and have a decidedly higher fatality. Older infants and adults seem to be less susceptible; most other bacterial and viral diseases producing diarrhea in the newborn also affect adults. No known means to induce immunity artificially.

8. *Occurrence.*—Frequent in North America and Europe, and probably more widespread than reports from other countries indicate. Primarily a disease of hospitals caring for newborn infants in nurseries. No definite seasonal incidence.

9. *Methods of control.*—Current practice is empirical, with principal dependence on general measures for limiting spread of infection and for conduct of a clean nursery.

    A. Preventive measures:

        1. A hospital nursery for the newborn or premature should accommodate no more than 12 infants; should not communicate directly with other nurseries; have at least 24 square feet of floor space per infant; and provide mechanically controlled running hot and cold water for hand washing. A "suspect" nursery should be provided to which infants can be transferred on the slightest suspicion of illness. Infants with established illness should be transferred to a separate isolation nursery or to the pediatric service. Because of the ease with which the

infection spreads, once introduced into a nursery, the increasing practice of keeping each baby with its mother has much to recommend it.

2. Individual equipment, kept at the bassinet, should be provided each infant; no common bathing or dressing tables and no bassinet stands for holding or transporting more than one infant at a time.

3. No nurse to care for more than 12 infants and their equipment, such care to be given at the bedside.

4. Feeding formulas, including glucose-water, should be prepared aseptically, placed in clean bottles with clean nipples attached and covered with a cap. The entire product should be subjected to terminal heating, either by steam under pressure 15 lbs. at 121.1° C. (250° F.) for 5 minutes, or 6 lbs. at 110° C. (230° F.) for 10 minutes) or by flowing steam, 100° C. (212° F.) for 30 minutes; then refrigerated with nipple caps left on bottles until feeding time. Periodic bacteriological sampling of heated formulas is recommended; coliform organisms should be absent and the total plate count should not exceed 10 organisms per ml.

5. Normal newborn infants should not be kept in the same nursery with sick infants or older children. An infant born outside the hospital or to a mother who has diarrheal or respiratory illness should not be admitted to the nursery for well infants except after isolation for at least four days, preferably with stool examination for potential pathogens. Nurses caring for patients should have no association with nurseries for normal newborn or premature infants; nurses engaged in the milk kitchen should not attend the infants' toilet; control of visitors to minimize spread of infection; laundry procedures to assure absence of pathogenic organisms from finished product as returned to nursery.

6. Systematic daily record of number and consistency of stools for each infant.

B. Control of the infected individual, contacts and environment:

1. Report to local health authority: Obligatory report of epidemics; no individual case report, Class 4 (p. 7). Two or more concurrent cases in a nursery are to be interpreted as an epidemic.

2. Isolation: Of infected infant, also suspects.

3. Concurrent disinfection: Of all discharges and articles soiled therewith.

4. Terminal disinfection: Thorough cleaning of nursery and equipment.

5. Quarantine: Complete quarantine of all newborn contacts.

6. Immunization: None.

7. Investigation of contacts and source of infection: See 9C2.

8. Specific treatment: The tetracycline antibiotics, chloramphenicol or sulfadiazine have been used in illnesses due to coliform group; and more recently, neomycin.

C. Epidemic measures:

1. Permit no new admissions to the contaminated hospital nursery; suspend maternity service unless uninfected nurseries with separate personnel and facilities are available. Exposed babies in the contaminated nursery should be cared for by separate medical and nursing personnel skilled in care of communicable disease; observe contacts for at least 2 weeks after last case leaves the nursery; promptly remove each new case to isolation. Maternity service may be resumed after discharge of all contact babies and mothers and thorough cleaning. Put into practice recommendations of 9A so far as feasible in the emergency.

2. Epidemiologic investigation: (a) Assure adequate treatment of missed cases by follow-up examination of all infants discharged from hospital during 2 weeks preceding first recognized case; (b) examine mothers and maternity service personnel for early signs of illness; (c) bacteriologic examination of feces of all sick and exposed babies, mothers and maternity service personnel to detect missed cases and carriers due to a known pathogen; (d) survey hospital for sanitary hazards; (e) investigate preparation of feeding formulas for adequacy of sterilization and refrigeration; bacteriologic examination of solutions and sugars used in formulas and their storage; bacteriologic examination of rubber nipples and bottle caps; (f) inquiry into technic of aseptic nursing of infants, of changing diapers, and of laundering diapers and other clothing.

D. International measures: None.

DIPHTHERIA

1. *Identification.*—An acute febrile infection, generally of tonsils, throat, and nose, marked by a patch or patches of grayish membrane from which the diphtheria bacillus is readily cultured. Occasionally, and especially in adults, there is only slight inflammation with little or no membrane. Inapparent infections of the upper respiratory tract outnumber recognized cases. Nasal diphtheria is commonly marked by one-sided nasal discharge and excoriated nares. Non-respiratory forms include infection of skin and wound surfaces; rarely the vagina. Cutaneous diphtheria usually appears as localized punched-out ulcers. Late effects of absorption of toxin include cranial nerve palsies and myocarditis. Fatality is variable; in some epidemics 10 to 12%, and commonly 2 to 5%.

Diagnosis is by clinical symptoms with confirmation by bacteriologic examination of discharges. Failure to demonstrate the bacillus in suspected diphtheria is not a valid reason for withholding specific treatment.

2. *Etiologic agent.*—Corynebacterium diphtheriae, the Klebs-Loeffler bacillus.

3. *Source and reservoir of infection.*—Discharges and secretions from mucous surfaces of nose, pharynx and nasopharynx of infected persons, and from skin and other lesions.

4. *Mode of transmission.*—Contact with a patient or carrier or with articles soiled with discharges of such persons. Milk has served as a vehicle.

5. *Incubation period.*—Usually 2 to 5 days, occasionally longer.

6. *Period of communicability.*—Variable, until virulent bacilli have disappeared from secretions and lesions; usually 2 weeks or less, seldom more than 4 weeks.

7. *Susceptibility and resistance.*—Infants born of immune mothers are relatively immune, a passive protection usually lost by the 6th month; in North America, probably not more than half of the mothers are immune. Recovery from an attack of the disease is usually but not necessarily followed by persisting immunity. Immunity is often acquired through unrecognized infection. Passive temporary immunity of 10 days to 3 weeks and active immunity of prolonged duration can be induced artificially.

8. *Occurrence.*—Endemic and epidemic; a disease of autumn and winter months. In communities where active immunization has been neglected, approximately one-fourth of cases and one-half of deaths occur in children under 5 years of age. In communities where childhood immunization has been adequate but reinforcing doses of toxoid were not continued, age distribution tends toward older persons. Clinical disease is more common in temperate zones than in the tropics, although infection rates are often much the same. Relatively, the tropics have more inapparent infection, less faucial diphtheria and more diphtheria of the skin.

9. *Methods of control:*

    A. Preventive measures:

        1. The only effectual control of diphtheria is through active immunization on a population basis. All children should be inoculated with diphtheria toxoid. The following procedure is recommended: at 2 to 6 months of age two adequate doses of diphtheria alum toxoid alone or combined with tetanus toxoid, 4 to 8 weeks apart; or three doses of combined pertussis vaccine and diphtheria toxoid (with or without added tetanus toxoid) administered at 3 to 5 week intervals; or 3 doses of fluid toxoid. Whether with toxoid alone or combined, the basic course of inoculations must be reinforced by at least one recall or "booster" dose within 3 to 12 months. Reinforcing doses are essential in pre-school life, desirable on entrance to school, and elective through school life and early adulthood. Where protection has been neglected in infancy, the program should be carried through as soon as the opportunity arises.

        2. Adults subject to unusual risk such as physicians, teachers, nurses, nursemaids, orderlies and other hospital personnel, should receive diphtheria toxoid. It is desirable to identify susceptibles by a Schick test (0.1 ml intradermally containing 0.001 Lf of stabilized nonphenolized toxin). In order to serve as an adequate control of the

Schick test and to reduce the hazard of severe local and constitutional reactions, an intradermal toxoid reaction test (0.1 cc of a 1 : 100 dilution fluid toxoid in saline solution) is recommended. Schick positive non-reactors to the control may be given toxoid in the usual dosage; persons who are Schick positive and also reactors should be given small doses of suitably diluted purified toxoid containing a minimal amount of alum.

3. A majority of young adults of military age become Schick negative in the course of protection against tetanus, when inoculated with a special preparation containing diphtheria toxoid (about 2 Lf) in each 1 cc of tetanus toxoid.

4. Pasteurization of milk supply.

5. Educational measures to inform the public and particularly the parents of little children of the hazards of diphtheria and the necessity and advantages of active immunization.

B. Control of the infected individual, contacts and environment:

1. Report to local health authority: Case report obligatory in most states and countries, Class 2A (p. 7).

2. Isolation: Until two cultures from throat and two from nose taken not less than 24 hours apart fail to show diphtheria bacilli. Local or general application of antibiotic or chemotherapeutic agents invalidates the usefulness of bacteriological examination. Isolation may be terminated if the microorganism reported present is proved avirulent. Where termination of case by culture is impracticable, isolation may end with fair safety 14 days after onset. Where practicable, a virulence test should be made if throat cultures are reported positive 3 weeks or more after onset.

3. Concurrent disinfection: Of all articles in contact with patient, and all articles soiled by discharges of patient.

4. Terminal disinfection: Thorough airing and sunning of the sick room, with cleaning.

5. Quarantine: All intimate contacts, especially young children, should be kept under surveillance if found to be carriers or suffering from nasal discharge or sore throat. Adult contacts whose occupation involves handling of food or close association with children should be excluded from these occupations until shown not to be carriers by bacteriological examination.

6. Immunization: Child contacts less than 10 years of age, intimately exposed and not previously immunized with toxoid, may be given a prophylactic dose of antitoxin, 10,000 units, and at the same time a first dose of toxoid. Daily examination by a physician is advised for older children and adults, with such further active immunization as may be indicated; persons previously immunized should have a reinforcing dose of toxoid. Groups of persons, as in institutions, barracks, or in closely congested quarters should have immediate Schick test, with toxoid reaction test, followed by active immunization of Schick positives.

7. Investigation of contacts and source of infection: Search for unreported and atypical cases, carriers, and contaminated milk.

8. Specific treatment: If diphtheria is suspected, antitoxin should be given without awaiting bacteriological confirmation. The earlier antitoxin is given the more effective it is: 20,000 to 80,000 units depending upon duration of symptoms, area of involvement, and severity of the disease; and in a single dose after completion of sensitivity tests. Intramuscular administration usually suffices; in severe infection antitoxin both intravenously and intramuscularly is indicated. Bed rest is essential to minimize the hazard of cardiac and other complications. Sulfonamides are of no value. Penicillin may be used in conjunction with antitoxin but is *not* a substitute for antitoxin. Neither penicillin nor diphtheria antitoxin can be relied upon to shorten materially the period of communicability. Penicillin soaked compresses (500 units per cc) are of value in cutaneous diphtheria; also erythromycin and bacitracin.

C. Epidemic measures:

1. Immediate intensification of efforts to provide artificial immunization by diphtheria toxoid to the largest possible numbers of the population affected, with first and greatest emphasis upon protection of infants and preschool children.

D. International measures:

1. Active immunization of susceptible infants and young children travelling to or through countries where diphtheria is a common disease; a reinforcing dose of toxoid for those previously inoculated.

2. Exchange of information between countries on current prevalence of diphtheria.

DIPHYLLOBOTHRIASIS

1. *Identification.*—An intestinal infection of man by an adult cestode. Symptoms are commonly trivial or absent. Some patients develop severe anemia; massive infections may be associated with toxic symptoms. A non-fatal infection of long duration. Synonym: Broad or Fish Tapeworm Infection.

Diagnosis is confirmed by identification in feces of proglottides (segments) of the worm, of scolex or of eggs.

2. *Etiologic agent.*—Diphyllobothrium latum, infection of man with adult worm only.

3. *Source and reservoir of infection.*—The immediate source of infection is the flesh of infected fresh water fish; the reservoir is feces of infected persons containing eggs. A number of other reservoir hosts including the dog and fish-eating mammals are relatively unimportant.

4. *Mode of transmission.*—Man acquires the infection by eating parasitized fish, raw or inadequately cooked. Larvae developing in flesh of freshwater fish are infective for definitive hosts. Eggs discharged from segments of worm must reach bodies of fresh water in which they mature, hatch, and produce infection in first intermediate host (Copepods). Susceptible fish in turn ingest infected Copepods and become second intermediate hosts.

5. *Incubation period.*—Five to six weeks.

6. *Period of communicability.*—Not transmissible from man to man. Man and other definitive hosts continue to disseminate eggs in the environment as long as the worm remains in the intestine, possibly for several years.

7. *Susceptibility and resistance.*—Man is universally susceptible. No apparent resistance follows infection.

8. *Occurrence.*—Endemic in Finland, Baltic states, Russia, Siberia, Switzerland, Israel, Japan, Uganda, North America (Great Lakes region, Eastern Canada, and Florida) and Chile, South America. In some areas 10 to 15% of the population are infected, prevalence increasing with age. Persons in the United States commonly of foreign origin and resident in cities, become infected from eating or sampling uncooked infected fish from Middle West lakes.

9. *Methods of control:*

   A. Preventive measures:
      1. Prevention of stream and lake pollution by installation of disposal systems for human discharges in cities and villages, by chlorination of sewage effluents, by sanitary privies in rural areas, and by education of the public.
      2. Thorough cooking of fish or freezing for twenty-four hours at $-10°$ C. insures protection. Inspection of fish is not practical.

   B. Control of the infected individual, contacts and environment:
      1. Report to local health authority: Official report not ordinarily justifiable, Class 5 (p. 7).
      2. Isolation: None.
      3. Concurrent disinfection: None; sanitary disposal of feces.
      4. Terminal disinfection: None.
      5. Quarantine: None.
      6. Immunization: None.
      7. Investigation of contacts and source of infection: Not usually a profitable procedure.
      8. Specific treatment: Oleoresin of aspidium or quinacrine.

   C. Epidemic measures: None.

   D. International measures: None.

DRACONTIASIS

1. *Identification.*—Infection with the nematode Dracunculus medinensis. The gravid female worm is about 1 meter long; it migrates to subcutaneous tissue, usually of the leg. First manifestation of infection is when gravid female prepares to discharge larvae from uterus located at anterior end; burning and itching sensation at the point of exit, and frequently nausea, vomiting, diarrhea, dyspnea and generalized urticaria. Eosinophilia is usual. A vesicle forms at the point of exit, ruptures; uterus of worm protrudes and discharges milky fluid containing larvae. Careless attempts to extract the worm before uterus is empty may result in secondary bacterial infection. A non-fatal disease other than for septic complications. Synonym: Guinea Worm Disease.

   Diagnosis is by microscopic identification of larvae or recognition of the adult worm after removal.

2. *Etiologic agent.*—Dracunculus medinensis, a nematode worm.

3. *Source and reservoir of infection.*—Water contaminated with infected Cyclops is immediate source of infection; reservoir is an infected person, through a worm discharging larvae from the skin.

4. *Mode of transmission.*—Larvae discharged into fresh water are swallowed by crustacea of the genus Cyclops; they penetrate into the body cavity and develop to the infective stage. Man swallows the Cyclops in drinking water, the larvae are liberated in the stomach or duodenum, migrate through the viscera, become adult and reach the subcutaneous tissues.

5. *Incubation period.*—From swallowing of infected Cyclops to onset of symptoms is about 8 to 14 months.

6. *Period of communicability.*—Until larvae have been completely evacuated from the uterus of the gravid worm; requires several days or weeks. Larvae may survive in water up to 6 weeks.

7. *Susceptibility and resistance.*—Susceptibility is general. Acquired immunity is non-existent; multiple and repeated infections occur in the same person.

8. *Occurrence.*—In India, Pakistan, Afghanistan, Russian Turkestan, Arabia, Iran, North and Central Africa, West Indies and the Guianas. Local prevalence varies greatly; in some localities nearly all inhabitants are infected, in others very few. In North America, worms morphologically identical to D. medinensis occur in dogs, foxes, mink and raccoons; no authentic indigenous case reported in man.

9. *Methods of control:*

   A. Preventive measures:
      1. Provision of potable water. Abolition of step-wells and other measures to prevent contamination of drinking water by infected persons through immersion of affected parts.
      2. Boiling of drinking water, or filtration through muslin cloth to remove Cyclops.
      3. Incomplete control of Cyclops can be had by treatment of wells with perchloron and copper sulfate, or by introducing a fish, Barbus puckelli or other species, which will destroy the intermediate host.

4. Education of the public to drink only boiled or filtered water. Instruction of infected persons in the mode of spread of the infection and the danger that exists in contaminating wells or other water supplies.

B. Control of the infected individual, contacts and environment:
  1. Report to local health authority: In selected endemic areas; in most countries not a reportable disease, Class 3C (p. 7).
  2. Isolation: None.
  3. Concurrent disinfection: None.
  4. Terminal disinfection: None.
  5. Quarantine: None.
  6. Immunization: None.
  7. Investigation of source of infection: Information should be obtained as to source of drinking water at probable time of infection. Locality should be searched for other cases, and sources of drinking water should be examined microscopically for infected Cyclops.
  8. Specific treatment: None.

C. Epidemic measures: In hyperendemic situations field survey to determine prevalence, investigation to discover sources of infection, and institution of control measures as in 9A.

D. International measures: None.

DYSENTERY, AMEBIC

1. *Identification.*—Amebic infection has a wide range of clinical manifestations. The primary site is the colon; infection may be asymptomatic, or with mild symptoms that include abdominal discomfort and diarrhea alternating with constipation, or a chronic diarrhea with mucus and some blood, or an acute dysentery with profuse blood and mucus, usually with little pus. Amebiasis is only occasionally a direct cause of death. Infection may spread by the blood stream or by direct extension, producing amebic hepatitis, abscess of liver, lung or brain, or ulceration of skin. Synonym: Amebiasis.

   Definitive diagnosis is through identifying trophozoites or cysts of Endamoeba histolytica in the feces, or trophozoites in smears or sections from lesions.

   Differential diagnosis includes shigellosis, appendicitis, and ulcerative colitis. Other intestinal protozoa are associated with diarrhea in man. Balantidiasis, caused by the ciliate protozoan Balantidium coli usually produces abdominal discomfort and a watery or mucoid diarrhea; sometimes severe ulceration of the colon similar to amebic dysentery. Giardia lamblia, an intestinal flagellate inhabiting the duodenum, is often associated with epigastric discomfort and mucoid diarrhea (giardiasis); both may exist concomitantly with E. histolytica.

2. *Etiologic agent.*—Endamoeba histolytica.

3. *Source and reservoir of infection.*—Cysts from feces of infected persons, usually chronic or asymptomatic cases. Acute infections are of little menace because of fragility of trophozoites.

4. *Mode of transmission.*—Contaminated vegetables, especially those commonly served raw, cold and moist; contaminated water; flies; soiled hands of infected food handlers.

5. *Incubation period.*—From 5 days in severe infections to several months in subacute and chronic cases; commonly 3 to 4 weeks.

6. *Period of communicability.*—During intestinal infection, which may be years if unrecognized and untreated.

7. *Susceptibility and resistance.*—Susceptibility to infection is general; relatively few persons harboring the organism develop recognized symptoms; acute cases tend to become chronic. Immunity to reinfection is not recognized in man. No artificial immunity.

8. *Occurrence.*—Distribution is world wide. Prevalence of infection is 50% or more in some unsanitated areas, especially in populations of moist tropics and in mental institutions; low (1 to 5%) in well sanitated cities. Foreigners entering tropical regions are particularly liable to acute dysenteric attack.

9. *Methods of control:*

   A. Preventive measures:

   1. Sanitary disposal of human feces.

   2. Protection of public water supplies against fecal contamination, and boiling drinking water where necessary. Chlorination of water supplies as generally practiced is inadequate for destruction of cysts; sand filtration removes nearly all cysts, diatomaceous earth filters completely. Avoidance of cross-connections between public and private auxiliary water supplies and of back-flow connections in plumbing systems. Small quantities of water, as in Lyster bags and canteens, are best protected by tablets of tetraglycine hydroperiodide (globaline).

   3. Supervision of general cleanliness, personal health, and sanitary practices of persons preparing and serving food in public eating places, especially moist foods eaten raw. Routine examination of food-handlers as a control measure is impractical.

   4. Disinfectant dips for fruits and vegetables are as yet of unproved value.

   5. Fly control and protection of foods against fly contamination by screening or other appropriate measure.

   6. Instruction of convalescents and of the general public in personal hygiene, particularly as to sanitary disposal of feces, and hand washing after defecation and before preparing or eating food.

   B. Control of the infected individual, contacts and environment:

   1. Report to local health authority: In selected endemic areas; in many states and countries not a reportable disease, Class 3C (p. 7).

   2. Isolation: None. Exclusion of patient from food preparation, processing, and serving.

   3. Concurrent disinfection: Sanitary disposal of feces. Hand washing after defecation.

   4. Terminal disinfection: Cleaning.

   5. Quarantine: None.

   6. Immunization: None.

7. Investigation of contacts and source of infection: Microscopic examination of feces of members of household, and of other suspected contacts, supplemented by search for direct contamination of water and foods by human feces.

8. Specific treatment: Acute amebic dysentery: Oxytetracycline (terramycin) is the drug of choice, with a relapse rate of 5 to 10%. Chlortetracycline (aureomycin) and chloramphenicol control the acute disease but relapse is more frequent. Emetine hydrochloride will relieve symptoms, but will usually not eliminate the intestinal infection; should be accompanied or followed by carbarsone, chiniofon, vioform or diodoquin. Some patients with ulceration of lower colon and rectum may require retention enemas of carbarsone or chiniofon.

Symptomless intestinal infections usually require no therapy.

Amebic hepatitis and liver abscess: chloroquin or emetine hydrochloride. If abscess requires drainage, precede by chloroquin or emetine to limit infection.

Repeated fecal examination at intervals up to six months is necessary to assure that pathogenic amebae have been eliminated.

C. Epidemic measures: Any grouping of several cases from a single area requires prompt epidemiologic investigation to determine source of infection and mode of transmission. If a common vehicle is indicated, such as water or food, take appropriate measures to correct the situation. Food handlers should be investigated, and if found infected, removed from duty. If the epidemiologic evidence points to person-to-person transmission, the emphasis is on sanitary disposal of feces, personal cleanliness and fly control.

D. International measures: None.

DYSENTERY, BACILLARY

1. *Identification.*—An acute bacterial infection characterized by diarrhea, fever, tenesmus and in severe cases blood and mucus in stool. Many patients with mild undiagnosed infections have only transient diarrhea or no intestinal symptoms. Severe infections are most frequent in infants, in elderly debilitated persons and in persons infected with Shiga bacillus; under other circumstances, the disease is rarely fatal. Synonym: Shigellosis.

Bacteriological diagnosis is by isolation of dysentery bacilli from feces or rectal swabs.

2. *Etiologic agent.*—Various species of genus Shigella (dysentery bacilli), Sonne, Flexner, Shiga and others.

3. *Source and reservoir of infection.*—Feces of infected persons. Many inapparent, mild and unrecognized infections.

4. *Mode of transmission.*—By eating contaminated foods, or drinking contaminated water or milk, and by hand-to-mouth transfer of contaminated material; by flies; by objects soiled with feces of a patient or carrier.

5. *Incubation period.*—One to 7 days, usually less than 4.

6. *Period of communicability.*—During acute infection and until microorganism is absent from feces, usually within a few weeks even without specific therapy; with some strains of shigella a few individuals become carriers for a year or two, rarely longer.

7. *Susceptibility and resistance.*—Susceptibility is general but disease is more common and more severe in children than in adults. A relative and transitory strain-specific immunity follows recovery.

8. *Occurrence.*—More common in United States than generally recognized; a high proportion of unreported diarrheas are dysentery. In England, Sonne infection is responsible for 90% of recognized cases; in United States, distributions of Flexner and Sonne strains are nearly equal. Shiga infection is rare in United States and Europe. Institutional outbreaks are frequent, with spread apparently by direct contact with unrecognized cases, or indirectly through nursing procedures and sometimes by food. In many parts of the world, especially the Orient, tropics and subtropics, dysentery is a common and serious infection, occurring at all ages and causing many deaths, particularly of small children.

9. *Methods of control:*

    A. Preventive measures:

        1. Sanitary disposal of human feces.

        2. Sanitary supervision of processing, preparation and serving of all foods, particularly those moist and eaten raw; special attention to provision and use of hand washing facilities.

        3. Boiling of milk or pasteurization of milk and dairy products.

        4. Persons suffering from diarrhea should be excluded from handling food for public consumption, and from handling family food supply if possible.

        5. Fly control and control of fly breeding; screening to protect foods against fly contamination.

        6. Protection and purification of public water supplies and construction of safe private supplies.

        7. Reduction of infant mortality in areas with high rates usually depends upon prevention of intestinal infection. Attention to the hygiene of breast feeding, scrupulous cleanliness in preparation, handling and refrigeration of food for children, boiling of milk for infant feeding, and continuous supervision of diet will contribute much to this aim. All infantile diarrhea should be regarded as bacillary dysentery until proved otherwise by bacteriologic examination of feces.

    B. Control of the infected individual, contacts and environment:

        1. Report to local health authority: Case report obligatory in most states and countries, Class 2B (p. 7). Recognition and report of epidemics have more than usual importance in schools and institutions.

2. Isolation: During acute illness. Rigid personal precautions by attendants. Surveillance during carrier state, which is usually temporary, and prohibition from food handling.

3. Concurrent disinfection: Of feces and of articles soiled therewith. In communities with a modern and adequate sewage disposal system, feces can be disposed of directly into the sewer without preliminary disinfection.

4. Terminal disinfection: Cleaning.

5. Quarantine: Contacts should not be employed as food handlers during period of contact nor before repeated negative feces cultures are obtained.

6. Immunization: No known satisfactory method.

7. Investigation of contacts and source of infection: Search for unrecognized mild cases and convalescent carriers among contacts. For sporadic cases, such investigation is time consuming and gives meagre results.

8. Specific treatment: The tetracycline antibiotics (aureomycin, terramycin), chloramphenicol and streptomycin given parenterally lead to rapid relief of symptoms, marked reduction in numbers of bacilli in from 24 to 48 hours and freedom from infection within several days. Streptomycin orally is also effective, especially when combined with sulfadiazine. Sulfadiazine may be used alone when antibiotics are not available.

C. Epidemic measures:

1. Groups of cases of acute diarrheal disorder should always be reported to local health authority at once, even in absence of exact identification of the disease.

2. Investigation of food, water, and milk supplies, general sanitation, and search for unrecognized mild cases and carriers.

3. Reduction in incidence may be expected from prophylactic administration of chemotherapeutic and antibiotic agents (see 9B8), given orally under medical supervision to groups of persons exposed temporarily to high risk of infection.

D. International measures: None.

ECHINOCOCCOSIS

1. *Identification.*—A disease caused by the cysts (hydatids) which are formed in various tissues by the developing larvae of the tapeworm, Echinococcus granulosus. Liver and lung are most frequently involved, also kidney, pelvis, heart, bone and central nervous system. Symptoms are variable. Fatality depends on site of cysts; they may give no symptoms through life, or in vital areas cause death. Synonyms: Hydatidosis, Echinococciasis.

Diagnosis is difficult unless the probability of exposure to infection can be established. X-ray examination is helpful in unilocular hydatid cyst, especially within the thorax. If cysts rupture, search should be made for hooklets, scolices, and cyst membranes in sputum, vomitus, urine, feces, or discharges from a sinus.

Eosinophilia may be present. Precipitin, complement fixation, and intradermal tests are diagnostic aids. Confirmation is by examination of tissues obtained surgically or at autopsy.

2. *Etiologic agent.*—Echinococcus granulosus, dog tapeworm; somatic infection with larvae only (hydatid disease) in man and numerous natural hosts including sheep, cattle, pigs, moose, caribou and marsupials.

3. *Source and reservoir of infection.*—Feces containing eggs from carnivores infected with adult worms, especially the domestic dog, wolf, dingo, and to a lesser extent, other Canidae, which are the primary hosts. The larval form occurs in ruminants, swine, equines and monkeys. The dog-sheep-dog cycle is important in endemic areas; the disease can be maintained in wild life.

4. *Mode of transmission.*—By ingesting contaminated foods and drinking water, and by hand-to-mouth transfer of eggs through contact with objects soiled with dog feces containing eggs. Airborne infection by inhalation of eggs may be possible.

5. *Incubation period.*—Variable, several years.

6. *Period of communicability.*—Not transmissible from man to man or from one intermediate host to another. Dogs continue to disseminate ova as long as they harbor the worm in the intestine.

7. *Susceptibility and resistance.*—Man is universally susceptible. No apparent resistance follows infection.

8. *Occurrence.*—The disease is relatively common in South America, Alaska, eastern Australia, New Zealand, and Middle East countries, to a lesser extent in England and Central Europe. Hydatid infection is rare in man in the United States, but relatively frequent in the Indian population of Canada.

9. *Methods of control:*

A. Preventive measures:

1. Rigid control of slaughtering of herbivorous animals so that dogs do not have access to scraps of uncooked meat. Dogs are infected only by larval forms, hydatid cysts, in food mammals.

2. Licensing and periodic examination of dogs, with reduction in numbers so far as may be compatible with occupational requirements in areas of endemic prevalence. Mass antihelminthic treatment of dogs has been successful in Iceland and Argentina.

3. Education of school children and of the general public in the dangers of close association with dogs, and of the need for controlled slaughtering of animals.

4. Incineration of dead animals.

B. Control of the infected individual, contacts and environment:

1. Report to local health authority: In selected endemic areas; not a reportable disease in most states and countries, Class 3B (p. 7).

2. Isolation: None.

3. Concurrent disinfection: None.

4. Terminal disinfection: None.

5. Quarantine: None.

6. Immunization: None.

7. Investigation of contacts and source of infection: Examination of familial contacts for suspicious tumors. Search for source in dogs kept in and about the house, animals slaughtered and hides and wool handled.

8. Specific treatment: None.

C. Epidemic measures:

1. In areas of high endemic prevalence, periodic destruction of wild, vagrant and non-essential dogs. Thorough treatment with antihelminthics of all essential dogs of the community twice yearly.

2. Systematic clinical, roentgenographic and serologic examination in the schools and among farmers, hunters, workers in warehouses for animal products, and others having close association with dogs.

D. International measures: Coordinated programs entered into by neighboring countries where the disease is endemic, designed to control the infection in animals and the movement of dogs from known enzootic areas.

ENCEPHALITIS, ARTHROPOD–BORNE VIRAL

1. *Identification.*—A group of acute inflammatory diseases of short duration, involving parts of the brain, spinal cord and meninges. The signs and symptoms are similar but with variation in severity and rate of progress. Mild cases may resemble non-paralytic poliomyelitis. Severe infections usually have acute onset, high fever, meningeal signs, stupor, disorientation, coma, spasticity, tremors, convulsions occasionally in infants, and spastic but rarely flaccid paralysis. The Russian type frequently leads to paralysis and atrophy of shoulder girdle. Fatality ranges from 5 to 60%, that of Japanese B and Eastern Equine types being highest. Permanent sequelae are rare except in infants; no parkinsonism. Mild leucocytosis is usual; leucocytes in spinal fluid from 50 to 200, occasionally 1,000 or more in infants.

Specific identification is by demonstrated rise in antibody between early and late serum specimens; by neutralization, complement fixation or by hemagglutination inhibition. Virus may be isolated from the brain of fatal cases; histopathological changes are not specific for individual viruses.

These diseases require differentiation from encephalitic and non-paralytic forms of poliomyelitis, rabies, mumps meningoencephalitis, lymphocytic choriomeningitis, herpes encephalitis, post-vaccinal or postinfection encephalitis, bacterial, protozoal, leptospiral and fungal meningitides or encephalitides; also the von Economo type of encephalitis (encephalitis lethargica) of unknown etiology, a disease of frequent occurrence in the years just before and after 1920 but now rarely reported.

2. *Etiologic agent.*—Each form of the disease is caused by a specific virus —Eastern Equine, Western Equine, St. Louis, Venezuelan Equine, Japanese B, Murray Valley, Russian Spring-Summer, West Nile and others. Some are interrelated immunologically.

3. *Source and reservoir of infection.*—Wild and domestic birds are the principal reservoirs of infection in the United States; although serving as hosts, horses are not important, nor is man for types found in United States; an infected mosquito is the immediate source of infection for man. Rodents are the reservoirs for the Russian type and ticks the source of infection.

4. *Mode of transmission.*—By the bite of mosquitoes, except for Russian Spring-Summer type which is tick-borne. In western and central United States and in Canada, Culex tarsalis is believed the principal vector; C. tritaeniorhynchus in the Far East; Culiseta melanura strongly suspect in eastern United States. Genus and species elsewhere are undetermined.

5. *Incubation period.*—Usually 5 to 15 days.

6. *Period of communicability.*—Not directly transmissible from man to man. Virus is not demonstrable in blood of man after onset of disease except in Venezuelan and Russian types.

7. *Susceptibility and resistance.*—Susceptibility to clinical disease usually highest in infancy and old age; inapparent or undiagnosed infection is more common at other ages. Infection of any degree apparently results in homologous immunity but not to other types. In several Far Eastern areas most adults are immune to local strains by reason of mild or inapparent infections, and susceptibles are mainly children.

8. *Occurrence.*—Eastern and Western Equine and St. Louis types are recognized human infections in United States and Canada, in some Central and South American countries one or other or both, and also the Venezuelan Equine type. Japanese B type is present in Japan, Korea, China, Malaya, and a number of Pacific islands. Murray Valley type of Australia is probably the originally described Australian X disease. Russian Spring-Summer type occurs in both European and Siberian Russia. West Nile is found in parts of northeast Africa, the Middle East and India. Other types of virus have been reported from United States and elsewhere, but pathogenicity for man is ill defined. A disease of summer and early fall, commonly limited to areas and years of high sustained temperature and many mosquitoes; has persisted for successive years in hot, irrigated western valley regions of the United States; irregularly epidemic in dry farming areas of midwest, southwest, and east. Highest rates are in rural and suburban districts.

9. *Methods of control:*

   A. Preventive measures:

      1. Destruction of larvae and elimination of breeding places of known or suspected vector mosquitoes.
      2. Killing mosquitoes by space spraying of human habitations.
      3. Screening of sleeping and living quarters; when disease is present, use mosquito bed-nets.
      4. Avoid exposure to mosquitoes during hours of biting, or use repellents.
      5. Education of the public as to mode of spread and control.
      6. Immunization of persons at great risk (laboratory workers and others) with experimental formalinized vaccines; not recommended for general use and not available commercially.

    7. Passive protection of accidentally exposed laboratory workers, by human or animal immune serum.

B. Control of the infected individual, contacts and environment:

    1. Report to local health authority: Case report obligatory in most states of the United States and in some other countries, Class 2A (p. 7).

    2. Isolation: None. Virus not usually found in blood, secretions, or discharges during clinical manifestations.

    3. Concurrent disinfection: None.

    4. Terminal disinfection: None.

    5. Quarantine: None.

    6. Immunization: Of contacts, none.

    7. Investigation of contacts and source of infection: Search for missed cases and presence of vector mosquitoes; primarily a community problem (see 9C).

    8. Specific treatment: None.

C. Epidemic measures: Identification of cases among horses and recognition of other human cases in the community is of epidemiological value to indicate frequency of infection and areas involved.

D. International measures: Insecticide spray of airplanes from recognized areas of prevalence.

ENTEROBIASIS

1. *Identification.*—An exceedingly common non-fatal intestinal infection which usually produces no symptoms. If severe, may cause pruritus ani, with disturbed sleep and irritability, and local irritation from scratching. A variety of severe manifestations including appendicitis and salpingitis have been described, but their relationship is indefinite. Synonyms: Pinworm or Threadworm Infection.

    Diagnosis is by swabbing a cellophane tipped applicator over the perianal region and examining microscopically for eggs; the swab is best obtained in the morning before bathing or defecation.

2. *Etiologic agent.*—Enterobius vermicularis, an intestinal round worm infecting only man. Eggs are infective within a few hours after leaving the gastrointestinal tract. After ingestion, eggs hatch in the stomach and small intestine; young worms mature in lower small intestine, cecum and upper portions of colon. Gravid worms migrate to the rectum to discharge eggs on perianal skin; may migrate up genital tract of females and enter peritoneal cavity.

3. *Source and reservoir of infection.*—Clothing and bedding soiled with feces containing eggs; contaminated food. Reservoir is infected persons, particularly children.

4. *Mode of transmission.*—Infective eggs may be transferred by hand from anal region to mouth of the same host, or indirectly to same host or new hosts through contaminated food and other objects. Dustborne infection by inhalation is possible in contaminated households.

5. *Incubation period.*—The life cycle requires about two months. Infections ordinarily build up from successive reinfections and are not recognized until several months.

6. *Period of communicability.*—Infected persons are potential spreaders of infection as long as they harbor the parasites.

7. *Susceptibility and resistance.*—Susceptibility is universal. Differences in incidence and intensity of infection are due to differences in frequency of exposure. No apparent resistance to repeated infections.

8. *Occurrence.*—Distribution is world-wide. An estimated 20 percent of the general population of the United States are infected. Prevalence is highest in children of school age, next highest in those of preschool age, and lowest in adults except for mothers of infected children, who commonly have a high rate. Infection is characteristically familial. Crowding is an important factor; incidence is often high in institutions.

9. *Methods of control:*

A. Preventive measures:

1. Maintenance of clean facilities for defecation.
2. Insistence upon practice of personal hygiene of the toilet, particularly the washing of hands after defecation and always before eating or preparing food.
3. Reduction of overcrowding in living accommodations; adequate provision of toilets and privies.
4. Bathing with sufficient frequency to keep the body clean; use of clean underclothing, night clothes and bed sheets at frequent intervals.
5. Habits of nail biting and scratching bare anal area should be discouraged.

B. Control of the infected individual, contacts and environment:

1. Report to local health authority: Official report not ordinarily justifiable, Class 5 (p. 7). School authorities should be advised of school outbreaks.
2. Isolation: None.
3. Concurrent disinfection: Sanitary disposal of feces and washing of hands in soap and water after defecating and before eating. Change bed linen and underwear of infected person daily and boil to kill eggs.
4. Terminal disinfection: None.
5. Quarantine: None.
6. Immunization: None.
7. Investigation of contacts and source of infection: Each infected individual is a source of infection. All members of an infected family or institution should be examined.
8. Specific treatment: Gentian violet medicinal by mouth is the usual therapy. The tetracyclines and particularly terramycin recently have been reported as preferred. All members of a household should be treated simultaneously.

C. Epidemic measures: Outbreaks in schools and institutions require strict hygienic measures and cleanliness. Toilet seats should be washed daily with disinfectant. Control measures should include facilities for treatment.

D. International measures: None.

FASCIOLOPSIASIS

1. *Identification.*—An infection of the small intestine with the trematode or fluke, Fasciolopsis buski. Symptoms are from toxic absorption rather than direct blood destruction. Severity depends on number of worms and the general state of health; death is rare. The large flattened red worms attach to mucous membranes of the small intestine, particularly duodenum. Diarrhea of a non-dysenteric type usually alternates with constipation; vomiting and anorexia are frequent; with large numbers of worms acute intestinal obstruction may occur. Patients may show edema of face within 20 days after infection and of abdominal wall and legs; ascites is common. Eosinophilia is usual, and secondary anemia occasional.

   Diagnosis depends on finding worms or characteristic eggs in feces. Eggs, easily detected because of their large size, are in greatest number in the first part of formed stools; occasionally worms are vomited.

   Differentiation is required from eggs of Fasciola hepatica, the fluke commonly infecting the bile ducts of sheep, cattle and other ruminants throughout the world. The disease, fascioliasis, is frequently reported in man in Cuba.

2. *Etiologic agent.*—Fasciolopsis buski.

3. *Source and reservoir of infection.*—Aquatic plants eaten raw; in China, nuts of the red water-caltrop grown in enclosed ponds, and tubers of the so-called "water chestnut" are among the sources of infection to man, as the hull or skin is peeled off with the teeth and lips. Man, pig and dog are definitive reservoir hosts of adult flukes.

4. *Mode of transmission.*—Eggs passed in feces develop within 3 to 7 weeks under favorable conditions; miracidia hatch, penetrate snails (Segmentininae of the Planorbidae) as intermediate host; cercariae develop, are liberated and encyst on aquatic plants which transmit the infection to man. Period of development from infection of snail to development of encysted, infective metacercariae is 7 to 8 weeks.

5. *Incubation period.*—About 3 months, from ingestion of infective larvae until passage of eggs.

6. *Period of communicability.*—As long as viable eggs are discharged by patient; without treatment, probably for many years.

7. *Susceptibility and resistance.*—Susceptibility is general; in undernourished individuals the ill effects are pronounced.

8. *Occurrence.*—Widely distributed in the Orient, including Central and South China, Formosa, Bengal, Assam, Thailand, Tonkin, Annam, Sumatra and Borneo. Prevalence is often extremely high.

9. *Methods of control:*

   A. Preventive measures:
      1. Education of people in endemic areas regarding life cycle of the parasite.
      2. Treatment of nightsoil before use as fertilizer; chemical treatment (unslaked lime, 1 part to 1,000 parts of water) or long storage destroys eggs, as do drying, freezing or heating.

3. Drying the particular plants involved, or if eaten fresh, dipping them into boiling water for a few seconds; both methods kill metacercariae.

4. Destruction of snail intermediate hosts.

B. Control of the infected individual, contacts and environment:

1. Report to local health authority: In selected endemic areas; in most countries not a reportable disease, Class 3C (p. 7).

2. Isolation: None.

3. Concurrent disinfection: Sanitary disposal of feces.

4. Terminal disinfection: None.

5. Quarantine: None.

6. Immunization: None.

7. Investigation of contacts and source of infection: Of the individual case, of little value. A community problem (see 9C).

8. Specific treatment: Hexylresorcinol crystoids (caprokol) has been used with considerable success.

C. Epidemic measures: Locate aquatic plants eaten fresh, which carry encysted metacercariae; identify infected snails in water with plants and prevent access of human feces to the water.

D. International measures: None.

FILARIASIS

1. *Identification.*—A nematode infection with early acute manifestations of fever, lymphadenitis, retrograde lymphangitis of extremities, orchitis, epididymitis, funiculitis and abscess. These are primarily allergic reactions, but secondary bacterial infection may occur and lead to the occasionally recorded death. After prolonged or repeated infection, obstruction to lymph flow often leads to hydrocele and elephantiasis of limbs, genitalia or breasts, or to chyluria. Female worms give rise to larvae, microfilariae, which in the absence of lymphatic obstruction, reach the blood stream. Many infected persons have no clinical manifestations but do have circulating microfilariae; many persons with clinical manifestations do not have circulating microfilariae. A nocturnal periodicity of microfilariae in the peripheral blood (10 p.m.–2 a.m.) occurs in all endemic areas except in those Pacific Islands where Aedes mosquitoes are the vectors.

Microfilariae are best detected in blood specimens taken at optimum time of day, and examined in thick-film preparation, or in stained sediment of laked blood. Skin test is non-specific and experimental.

Other filarial infections within an endemic area require differentiation, such as loaiasis (Loa loa) in central West Africa.

2. *Etiologic agents.*—Nematode worms, Wuchereria bancrofti and W. malayi.

3. *Source and reservoir of infection.*—Source is a mosquito; reservoir is blood of an infected person bearing microfilariae.

4. *Mode of transmission.*—By bite of mosquitoes harboring infective larvae. W. bancrofti is transmitted in nature by many species, the most important Culex fatigans, C. pipiens, Aëdes polynesiensis (pseudoscutellaris), and several species of Anopheles. W. malayi is transmitted by several species of Mansonia and Anopheles. The microfilariae penetrate the stomach wall of the mosquito, lodge in thoracic muscles, develop into infective larvae, migrate to the proboscis, and are transmitted to the new host as the infected mosquito bites.

5. *Incubation period.*—Allergic manifestations may appear as early as 3 months after infection. Microfilariae do not appear in the blood until at least 9 months.

6. *Period of communicability.*—In man, as long as microfilariae are present in the blood, which may be years. In the mosquito, from at least 10 days after infective feed until all infective larvae have been discharged or mosquito dies.

7. *Susceptibility and resistance.*—All persons are probably susceptible. Repeated infection apparently occurs in endemic regions. Acquired immunity is unknown.

8. *Occurrence.*—W. bancrofti is endemic in the West Indies, coastal Central America, northern and eastern South America, Central and Northern Africa, a few small areas of southern Europe, Arabia, Madagascar, India, Southeast Asia, China, Korea, Japan, northern Australia, and most of the Pacific Islands. W. malayi is endemic only in southeast Asia, India, central China and a few islands of Indonesia. Local foci of high prevalence are often surrounded by non-endemic areas. High prevalence depends upon a large reservoir of infection and abundant vector breeding.

9. *Methods of control:*

    A. Preventive measures:

        1. Anti-mosquito measures. Determine by dissection the vector or vectors in each locality; study times and places of feeding and locate breeding places. Attack adult mosquitoes by residual spraying of buildings with an acceptable insecticide (DDT or other), screening of houses, use of bednets, and insect repellents. Attack larvae by eliminating small breeding places and treating others with larvicides. Each local situation requires individual study.

        2. Education of the public concerning mode of transmission, and methods of mosquito control.

    B. Control of the infected individual, contacts and environment:

        1. Report to local health authority: In selected endemic regions; in most countries not a reportable disease, Class 3C (p. 7). Reporting of cases with demonstrated microfilariae provides data on potential transmission. Cases of elephantiasis without microfilariae in the blood should not be reported as filariasis, but are usefully recorded in estimating prevalence or in planning control programs.

        2. Isolation: Not practicable. So far as possible patients with microfilariae in blood should be protected from mosquito bites as a means of reducing transmission.

        3. Concurrent disinfection: None.

4. Terminal disinfection: None.
5. Quarantine: None.
6. Immunization: None.
7. Investigation of contacts and source of infection: Only as a part of a general community effort. (See 9A and 9C).
8. Specific treatment: Diethylcarbamazine (hetrazan) results in rapid disappearance of most or all microfilariae from the blood, but may not kill or even sterilize the adult female worm; microfilariae reappear in most cases after several months. Sodium thiacetarsamide (Caparsolate sodium) causes slow disappearance of microfilariae during treatment without subsequent increase over a 2-year period. Action of this compound apparently is against adult worms rather than microfilariae.

C. Epidemic measures: The first essential in a program of control in areas of high endemicity is an appraisal of the local situation, particularly the bionomics of mosquito vectors, prevalence and incidence of disease, and environmental factors responsible for transmission. Vector control is the fundamental approach. Even partial control by anti-mosquito measures may reduce incidence of new infections and restrict the endemic focus. Measurable results are slow because of the long incubation period. Mass treatment of known infected persons by chemotherapy contributes materially.

D. International measures: Coordinated programs entered into by neighboring countries where the disease is endemic with the purpose of limiting migration of infected persons across international boundaries, and instituting treatment and other control measures near such boundaries.

FOOD POISONING

Food poisoning is a generic term for disease of man characterized by gastro-enteritis of abrupt evolution, acquired through food, having a characteristic grouping of cases, and arising either from intoxication or infection. Numerous organic and inorganic substances act as agents of intoxication, and a number of microorganisms as infectious agents. The interest here is in intoxications of bacterial origin, and in infections due to salmonella.

Food poisoning is distinguished from food-borne infection. The effects of food poisoning are promptly evident and the amount of the particular food ingested has a relation to severity, suggesting the importance of preformed elements. Food-borne infection, with a number of intestinal pathogens, with streptococci and with the agents of diphtheria, tuberculosis and undulant fever, follows a usual incubation for the particular disease, and clinical course and manifestations are not as a rule materially altered by the circumstance of food serving as the vehicle of infection.

A. Staphylococcus Intoxication

1. *Identification.*—A poisoning (not infection) of abrupt and sometimes violent onset with severe nausea, vomiting and prostration; sometimes severe diarrhea. Deaths are exceedingly rare. Diagnosis is

usually on the basis of grouping of cases and short interval between eating food and onset of symptoms.

Isolation of large numbers of staphylococci from suspected food permits presumptive diagnosis. Demonstration of ability of the organism to produce enterotoxin is essential for confirmation.

2. *Etiologic agent.*—Toxin (enterotoxin) of certain strains of staphylococci. The toxin is stable at boiling temperature; staphylococci multiply in food, producing toxin which causes poisoning.

3. *Source and reservoir of infection.*—(Not an infection but a poisoning.) Source of contamination not known in most instances; believed to be of human origin.

4. *Mode of transmission.*—Most common vehicle is custard-filled pastry; processed meats, especially ham, are responsible for some outbreaks; milk from cows with specifically infected udders.

5. *Incubation period.*—Interval between taking food and onset is one-half hour to 4 hours, usually 2 to 4.

6. *Period of communicability.*—Not applicable.

7. *Susceptibility and resistance.*—Most persons are susceptible, although individual reaction is variable.

8. *Occurrence.*—Widespread and a relatively frequent disease; staphylococcus infection is the principal cause of acute food poisoning in the United States.

9. *Methods of control:*

   A. Preventive measures:

   1. Prompt refrigeration of sliced and chopped meats and of custards and cream fillings, to avoid multiplication of staphylococci accidentally introduced; filling of pastries with custard immediately before sale, or adequate heat treatment of finished product. Avoid improper care of leftover foods.
   2. Some health departments have forbidden sale of custard-filled products during summer months.
   3. Temporary exclusion from food handling of persons suffering from pyogenic skin infections, especially of the hands.
   4. Education of food handlers in strict attention to sanitation and cleanliness of kitchens, including refrigeration, handwashing and the danger of working while having skin infections.

   B. Control of the infected individual, contacts and environment:

   1. Report to local health authority: Obligatory report of epidemics; also suspected or confirmed cases with evidence of grouping or association with others in time and place, Class 4 (p. 7).
   2. Isolation: None.
   3. Concurrent disinfection: None.
   4. Terminal disinfection: None.
   5. Quarantine: None.
   6. Immunization: None.
   7. Investigation of contacts and source of infection: Search for food contaminated with staphylococci, and for food handlers showing pyogenic skin infections or sore throat.
   8. Specific treatment: None.

C. Epidemic measures:

    1. Search for food contaminated with staphylococci and for food handlers with skin infections or sore throat.

    2. Destruction of any remainder of contaminated food after samples have been taken for laboratory examination.

D. International measures: None.

B. Botulinus Intoxication (Botulism)

1. *Identification.*—A highly fatal afebrile poisoning (not infection) characterized by headache, weakness, constipation, oculomotor or other paralysis and absence of diarrhea. Death by cardiac or respiratory paralysis occurs in about two-thirds of patients and usually within 3 to 7 days. Symptoms develop according to amount of toxin ingested in relation to body weight.

    Biologic and toxicologic tests may confirm presence of bacterium or its toxin in suspected food or stomach contents.

2. *Etiologic agent.*—Toxins produced by Clostridium botulinum or Cl. parabotulinum (botulinus bacillus). Most outbreaks are due to toxin from type A or B organisms; a few from type E. Toxin is produced in improperly processed food only under anaerobic conditions and particularly in non-acid foods. Toxin is easily destroyed by boiling but spores require higher temperatures.

3. *Source and reservoir of infection.*—Not an infection but a poisoning. The immediate source is food containing botulinus toxin. The reservoir of botulinus bacillus is soil and the intestinal tract of animals. Toxin is formed by anaerobic growth of spores in food.

4. *Mode of transmission.*—By ingestion of food containing botulinus toxin, usually eaten uncooked, and from jars or cans inadequately processed during canning. Most poisonings in the United States are due to home canned vegetables; in Europe most cases are due to sausages or other smoked or preserved meat.

5. *Incubation period.*—Symptoms usually appear within 18 hours after eating food containing toxin, possibly longer, the interval being determined by amount of contaminated food taken and content of botulinus toxin.

6. *Period of communicability.*—Not applicable.

7. *Susceptibility and resistance.*—Susceptibility is general.

8. *Occurrence.*—Sporadic and grouped cases occur in all countries and always in relation to some perishable food product which has been so kept or preserved as to permit botulinus bacilli to produce toxin.

9. *Methods of control:*

    A. Preventive measures:

        1. Governmental control by regulation and inspection of commercial processing of canned and preserved foods.

        2. Education of housewives and others concerned with home canning of foods, in essentials of safe processing, as to time, pressure and temperature factors.

        3. Education in value of boiling home canned green and leafy vegetables before serving; also thorough cooking of sausage and other meat and fish products.

B. Control of the affected (poisoned) individual, contacts and environment:
   1. Report to local health authority: Case report obligatory in most states and countries, Class 2A (p. 7). Includes suspect and confirmed cases.
   2. Isolation: None.
   3. Concurrent disinfection: None.
   4. Terminal disinfection: None.
   5. Quarantine: None.
   6. Immunization: Polyvalent botulinus antitoxin of appropriate type, if available, should be given to all who have eaten suspected food.
   7. Investigation of contacts and source of infection: Search for contaminated food. Study of food habits and recent food history of persons attacked.
   8. Specific treatment: Intramuscular administration of botulinus antitoxin.

C. Epidemic measures:
   1. Suspicion or recognition of a case of botulism should immediately raise question of a group outbreak. Single sporadic cases are uncommon.
   2. Immediate search for persons who shared suspected food, for persons who may have eaten comparable food from same source, and for any remaining food from same source that may be similarly contaminated, such food if found, to be destroyed after samples have been taken for laboratory examination. Search for limberneck in chickens.

D. International measures: None.

C. Salmonella Infection

1. *Identification.*—Salmonellosis includes a variety of clinical syndromes. The most common is an acute gastro-enteritis with diarrhea and abdominal cramps, to which attention is here limited. Fever, nausea and vomiting are frequently present. Deaths are uncommon but somewhat more frequent than for staphylococcal food poisoning.

   Salmonella may be recovered from feces or from the site of a localized infection during the acute illness, but isolation of the infectious agent is progressively more difficult during convalescence.

2. *Etiologic agent.*—Numerous species of Salmonella of the group pathogenic for animals and occasionally for man, and excluding primarily human pathogens (see Typhoid and Paratyphoid fevers, pp. 201, 117). Those more common in the United States are S. typhimurium, S. choleraesuis, S. newport, S. oranienburg, S. montevideo, S. panama and S. anatum; much variation from country to country; total serological types involved in food poisoning approach one hundred.

3. *Source and reservoir of infection.*—Feces of patients and convalescent carriers, especially mild and unrecognized infections. Feces of domestic fowl, household pets, rodents and domestic animals; eggs of ducks, less commonly of chickens.

4. *Mode of transmission.*—Epidemics are usually traced to (1) improperly prepared food, especially meat pies and roast fowl; (2) insufficiently

cooked foods containing dried hen eggs, or duck eggs; (3) unpasteurized milk or dairy products; (4) pastries contaminated by rodent feces, possibly through medium of cockroaches; (5) food prepared by an infected food handler. Sporadic cases probably originate through direct contact with an infected person or animal.

5. *Incubation period.*—In epidemics, 6 to 48 hours, usually about 12 hours. Not known for sporadic cases, but believed to be from 1 to 7 days.

6. *Period of communicability.*—Throughout infection. Extremely variable, usually 3 days to 3 weeks or as long as carrier state persists.

7. *Susceptibility and resistance.*—Susceptibility is general, with an apparently important relationship to size of infecting dose. No active or passive artificial immunization. Some species-specific immunity of brief duration probably follows recovery.

8. *Occurrence.*—World-wide and a common disease. Usually recognized in its epidemic form by groupings of cases among individuals having a common food supply. In such circumstances, a high proportion of individuals develop clinical symptoms. Sporadic cases tend to include more instances of mild unrecognized infection than of clinically evident disease.

9. *Methods of control:*

A. Preventive measures:

1. Thorough cooking of all foodstuffs derived from animal sources. Particular attention to preparation of fowl, egg products and meat dishes.
2. Protection of prepared food against rodent or insect contamination.
3. Refrigeration of prepared food during storage.
4. Attempts to control salmonella infection among domestic animals.
5. Meat and poultry inspection with adequate supervision of abattoir hygiene.

C. Control of the infected individual, contacts and environment:

1. Report to local health authority: Obligatory report of epidemics; also suspected or confirmed cases with evidence of grouping or association with others in time and place, Class 4 (p. 7).
2. Isolation: Exclusion of infected persons from food handling and occupations involving care of young children until negative feces cultures have been obtained.
3. Concurrent disinfection: Of feces and of articles soiled therewith. In communities with modern and adequate sewage disposal systems, feces can be disposed of directly into sewer without preliminary disinfection.
4. Terminal disinfection: Cleaning.
5. Quarantine: Family contacts should not be employed as food handlers during period of contact nor before repeated negative feces cultures have been obtained.
6. Immunization: None.
7. Investigation of contacts and source of infection: Search for unrecognized mild cases and convalescent carriers among contacts.
8. Specific treatment: None; chloramphenicol and the tetracycline antibiotics have limited and irregular effect.

C. Epidemic measures:
1. Intensive search for case or carrier who is source of infection.
2. Search for food which may have served as a vehicle of spread, attempt to determine method of contamination, and culture food bacteriologically.
3. Destruction of any remainder of suspected food after samples have been taken for laboratory examination.

D. International measures: An International Salmonella Center in Copenhagen, Denmark, and national salmonella centers in various countries (e.g., Communicable Disease Center, Atlanta, Ga., USA) facilitate proper identification of the various salmonella types. These centers provide uniformity of method and are essential to proper epidemiologic investigation of salmonellosis.

GLANDERS

1. *Identification.*—Glanders is a highly communicable disease of solipeds (horses, mules and donkeys), but rare in man. Two clinical forms occur, an infection of the skin known as farcy and a generalized infection known as glanders. Both may be acute or chronic, chronic infection being the more common in animals and acute infection in man. Infection of man may be clinical or inapparent; symptoms vary widely. Infections originating in the skin are characterized by appearance of a nodule at the site of inoculation, a surrounding area of lymphangitis and swelling, a generalized papular and sometimes pustular eruption, and bronchopneumonia; highly fatal, often within 8 to 10 days. Primary infections of nasal mucosa tend to resemble chronic glanders of the horse but are more often fatal, with ulcers of mucosa, regional lymphangitis and adenitis, and general dissemination of infection including skin lesions and joint manifestations. Laboratory infection through inhalation of infectious material produces pneumonitis resembling viral pneumonia.

Diagnosis is by complement fixation test, positive in the third week; agglutination test with rise in antibodies in the second week; late appearance of mallein reaction; and by bacteriological culture and isolation of the organism from lesions of experimentally infected hamsters and guinea pigs.

Melioidosis, a disease resembling glanders, is to be differentiated. Chief clinical features are septimemia and formation of characteristic granulomatous nodules in nearly all parts of the body. Caused by Malleomyces pseudomallei, with the natural reservoir in rats. Cases among American soldiers in World War II, Burma and Guam; reported in recent years in continental United States; countries of major frequency are Malay States, Indochina and Ceylon.

2. *Etiologic agent.*—Malleomyces mallei, glanders bacillus.

3. *Source and reservoir of infection.*—Discharges from open lesions of the respiratory tract or from exudates of skin lesions of infected horse or man.

4. *Mode of transmission.*—Infection in man is through inoculation of skin by direct contact with diseased animals, their tissues, cultures of

the organism, or in handling artificially infected laboratory animals; to a lesser extent by indirect contact with articles soiled with discharges. Hand-to-mouth transmission and infection by ingestion also occur. Rarely transmitted from man to man, among attendants caring for patients. Laboratory infections are relatively frequent, by inoculation of skin or airborne by inhalation of moist particles containing the infectious agent.

5. *Incubation period.*—Variable; usually one to five days.

6. *Period of communicability.*—Until organisms disappear from discharges or until lesions have healed.

7. *Susceptibility and resistance.*—Man apparently has a high grade inherent insusceptibility. Despite close association with animals where half or more are infected, cases in man are few. In this respect glanders is like foot and mouth disease, where authenticated infection in man is highly uncommon and existing ideas of frequency much overrated.

8. *Occurrence.*—Rare and sporadic; almost exclusively in occupations bringing contact with animals, such as stablemen, persons treating or conducting autopsies of glandered animals, and laboratory workers. Of decreasing world frequency as mechanized transport replaces horse drawn vehicles; still observed in many countries of Asia, Africa, Eastern Europe and South America. At long intervals cases are seen in North America and Western Europe.

9. *Methods of control:*

   A. Preventive measures:

      1. Prevention of glanders in man depends primarily upon control of glanders in equine species. In areas of endemic prevalence, measures include abolition of common feeding and drinking troughs for horses, sanitary supervision of stables and other places where horses are kept, and annual mallein testing of all horses and members of the horse family, also when offered for sale.

      2. Extreme care should be practiced by all laboratory workers handling cultures of this organism or artificially infected laboratory animals, their cages, and materials with which they have come in contact.

   B. Control of the infected individual, contacts and environment:

      1. Report to local health authority: Case report obligatory in most states and countries, Class 2A (p. 7). Report also to local livestock sanitary or agriculture authority.

      2. Isolation: At home or hospital; attendants should exercise scrupulous care to avoid contact with skin lesions or nasal secretions.

      3. Concurrent disinfection: Discharges from patients and articles soiled therewith.

      4. Terminal disinfection: Thorough cleaning.

      5. Quarantine: None.

      6. Immunization: No effective procedure.

      7. Investigation of contacts and source of infection: Human carriers are unknown. The problem is of animals (see 9C).

      8. Specific treatment: Experience is limited, but effective results are reported with sulfadiazine; penicillin or erythromycin may be useful.

C. Epidemic measures:
1. Not applicable to man, a sporadic disease.
2. Principal concern is with outbreaks among horses and other solipeds, which may be widespread or local. Quarantine of all animals in a contaminated stable until all have been mallein tested and retested, infected animals removed and stable, materials and surroundings disinfected. Destruction of infected animals is essential. Isolate newly arrived animals until freedom from glanders is assured by negative mallein test.

D. International measures: None.

GONOCOCCAL INFECTION

Urethritis and salpingitis of adults, vulvovaginitis of children and ophthalmia of newborn and adults are inflammatory conditions caused in common by gonococci. All are maintained in a population by reason of the continued presence of gonorrhea: together they constitute an epidemiologic entity and similar principles of control apply to the group. Clinically indistinguishable infections of the same anatomic structures are caused by a number of other infectious agents. This presentation relates specifically to gonococcal disease but the final paragraph under identification of each of the three gonococcal conditions gives the general characteristics of these other infections. They occur frequently and methods of control are often ill defined.

A. Gonococcal Urethritis (Gonorrhea)

1. *Identification.*—A more or less self-limited infectious disease of venereal origin initiated by the gonococcus, an organism having affinity for columnar and transitional epithelium. The disease is thereby limited to areas where such tissues are found. Accordingly, gonorrhea in the male and female differs in course, in seriousness and in ease of identification. In males, a thick yellow purulent discharge of the anterior urethra usually appears 3 to 9 days after effective exposure; infection may extend to the posterior urethra and after varying intervals result in epididymitis, prostatitis, arthritis, and endocarditis. In females, the disorder is in three stages: (1) a few days after exposure, an initial urethritis or cervicitis, often so mild as to pass unnoticed; (2) a stage of pelvic invasion, usually accompanying the first, second, or later menstrual period after infection, with mild or severe symptoms of salpingitis or pelvic peritonitis; (3) a stage of residual and often chronic infection. Death from gonorrhea is rare, but early and late manifestations, especially complications, are commonly and seriously incapacitating.

Bacteriologic culture is requisite to diagnosis of gonorrhea in the female, and desirable in gonorrhea of the male.

Widespread and frequent non-gonococcal urethritis, possibly also of sexual origin, seriously complicates the clinical diagnosis of gonorrhea in the male. In some countries the incidence exceeds that of gonorrhea and the condition is reportable. It is notoriously resistant to treatment, and much is unknown of etiology, communicability, clinical course and control; it may be initiated by a number of infectious agents.

2. *Etiologic agent.*—Neisseria gonorrhoeae, the gonococcus.

3. *Source and reservoir of infection.*—Exudate from mucous membranes of infected persons. Man is the only reservoir.

4. *Mode of transmission.*—Almost wholly by sexual intercourse, even in children; occasionally, in the newborn, by transfer from an ophthalmic infection acquired during birth; and in institutions for children, by careless and indiscriminate use of rectal thermometers.

5. *Incubation period.*—Usually 3 to 9 days, sometimes 14.

6. *Period of communicability.*—For months or years unless interrupted by specific therapy, which ends communicability within hours or days.

7. *Susceptibility and resistance.*—Susceptibility is general. Spontaneous recovery is usual in the absence of reinfection. Acquired immunity is not demonstrated; one attack does not protect against subsequent infection.

8. *Occurrence.*—Worldwide and a common disease, particularly among persons of lower economic status; affects both sexes and practically all ages, especially the age groups of greatest sexual activity. The decline in frequency of gonorrhea has not kept pace with that of syphilis; lack of accurate diagnosis and incomplete reporting preclude reliable estimates of incidence.

9. *Methods of control:*

A. Preventive measures:

1. Except for measures applying specifically to gonorrhea, primarily the use of chemoprophylactic agents in the eyes of the newborn (9A 1, p. 80) and special attention (abortive treatment) to female contacts of male patients (9B 7 infra), the preventive measures are those of Syphilis (see 9A, p. 178).

B. Control of the infected individual, contacts and environment:

1. Report to local health authority: Case report is required in many states and countries, Class 2B (p. 7).

2. Isolation: None; antibiotics promptly render discharges noninfectious. Refrain from sexual intercourse with untreated previous sexual partners to avoid reinfection.

3. Concurrent disinfection: Care in disposal of discharges from lesions and articles soiled therewith.

4. Terminal disinfection: None.

5. Quarantine: None.

6. Immunization: None.

7. Investigation of contacts and source of infection: Interview of patients and tracing of contacts are the fundamental features of a program for control. Trained interviewers obtain the best results. Female contacts of male patients with gonorrhea should be treated at once, on epidemiologic grounds only, because of delays and difficulties in diagnosis and the practical fact that sexual exposure continues despite advice to the contrary. Include all sexual contacts of ten days prior to onset; also examine serologically for syphilis over a period of several weeks.

8. Specific treatment: Procaine penicillin or bicillin in one intramuscular injection on clinical, laboratory or epidemiological grounds.

C. Epidemic measures: Intensification of routine procedures, especially therapy on epidemiologic grounds.

D. International measures: (See Syphilis 9D, p. 179).

B. Gonococcal Vulvovaginitis of Children

1. *Identification.*—An inflammatory reaction of the urogenital tract of prepubescent females, characterized by redness and swelling of mucous membrane and mucopurulent discharge of varying degree; in severe infections, excoriation of labia and thighs and extension to urethra and bladder. A self-limited disease in that more than three-fourths of patients recover spontaneously within 3 to 6 months; a carrier state sometimes persists.

Diagnosis is established by bacteriologic culture of exudates; stained smears are unreliable.

Gonococcal vulvovaginitis is to be differentiated from acute vulvovaginitis due to a variety of other infectious agents. In the United States, the gonococcus is responsible for only a small proportion (about 25%) of all cases. Clinical manifestations are usually indistinguishable and recognition is by bacteriological means. Outbreaks of non-gonococcal proctitis and vulvovaginitis occur in institutions for children.

2. *Etiologic agent.*—Neisseria gonorrhoeae, gonococcus.

3. *Source and reservoir of infection.*—Exudates from infected persons; infrequently, contaminated moist articles. The existence of transient inapparent gonococcus infection among children has been proven.

4. *Mode of transmission.*—Intimate direct contact with adult patients in the home, willing and unwilling sexual contact, and insertion of contaminated instruments and foreign bodies in vagina and rectum.

5. *Incubation period.*—Usually 3 to 9 days.

6. *Period of communicability.*—While discharges persist, usually 3 to 6 months; communicability may continue after clinical manifestations cease.

7. *Susceptibility and resistance.*—Susceptibility is related to type of epithelium lining vagina; until puberty: columnar or transitional epithelium; after puberty: stratified squamous type, not attacked by gonococci. Susceptibility is general among female children; the frequency of spontaneous recovery is proof of a developing resistance. One attack does not protect against subsequent infection.

8. *Occurrence.*—Extent not known but presumably widespread, particularly in families of lower social and economic levels where standards of personal, sexual, and general hygiene are low. Epidemics are most frequent in institutions for children.

9. *Methods of control:*

A. Preventive measures:

1. Fundamentally dependent on control of gonorrhea (see p. 77); general measures are those of Syphilis (see 9A, p. 178).

2. Proper supervision of institutions for children, with rigid enforcement of hygienic principles and realization that sex education must begin earlier in life than commonly believed.

B. Control of the infected individual, contacts and environment:

1. Report to local health authority: Case report is required in most states and countries, Class 2A (p. 7).

2. Isolation: For the first 24 hours after administration of antibiotics.

3. Concurrent disinfection: Care in disposal of discharges from lesions and articles soiled therewith.

4. Terminal disinfection: None.

5. Quarantine: None.

6. Immunization: None.

7. Investigation of contacts and source of infection: The proven importance of sexual transmission among children calls for trained interviewers to elicit history of sexual contact among playmates, family members and older males within the family group and outside. Histories are unreliable; actual search for gonorrhea among persons in the environment of the child is therefore necessary.

8. Specific treatment: Penicillin in a single repository dose.

C. Epidemic measures:

1. Prompt search for source of infection within the institution or group affected and introduction of measures to protect pre-adolescent and younger girl children.

2. Education of those in charge of children as to causes of outbreaks, and the sources and development of the disease, with special emphasis upon personal cleanliness of children. The importance of probable sexual transmission should be emphasized.

D. International measures: None.

C. Gonococcal Ophthalmia Neonatorum

1. *Identification.*—Acute redness and swelling of the conjunctiva of one or both eyes, with mucopurulent or purulent discharge in which gonococci are identifiable by microscopic and cultural methods.

Gonococcal ophthalmia neonatorum is but one of a number of acute inflammatory conditions of the eye or of the conjunctiva occurring within the first 3 weeks of life, and collectively known as ophthalmia neonatorum, acute conjunctivitis of the newborn, and babies' sore eyes of the first 21 days of life. Differentiation within the group is by bacteriologic means; clinical distinction is indefinite. The gonococcus is the most important but not necessarily the most frequent among infecting agents, which include meningococci, hemophilic bacilli, a virus (inclusion blenorrhea) and others. All purulent inflammation of the conjunctiva of the newborn is to be regarded as gonococcal until proved otherwise.

2. *Etiologic agent.*—Neisseria gonorrhoeae, gonococcus.

3. *Source and reservoir of infection.*—Infected maternal birth canal.

4. *Mode of transmission.*—Contact during childbirth.

5. *Incubation period.*—Usually 36 to 48 hours.

6. *Period of communicability.*—During the course of the disease and until discharges from infected membranes have ceased.

7. *Susceptibility and resistance.*—Susceptibility is general. Immunity to subsequent gonococcal infection does not follow attack.

8. *Occurrence.*—Varies widely according to observance or neglect of prophylactic use of a solution of silver nitrate or equivalent preparation in the eyes of the newborn by attendants at delivery. Infrequent where care of the newborn is adequate; globalwise, the disease is still an important cause of blindness.

9. *Methods of control:*

   A. Preventive measures:

   1. Specific protection by diagnosis and treatment of gonorrhea of the mother during prenatal period and installation of silver nitrate or equivalent preparation in the eyes of babies at birth.

   2. Depends fundamentally on control of gonorrhea (see p. 77); general preventive measures are those of Syphilis (see 9A, p. 178).

   B. Control of the infected individual, contacts and environment:

   1. Report to local health authority: Case report is required in most states and countries, Class 2A (p. 7).

   2. Isolation: For the first 24 hours after administration of antibiotic.

   3. Concurrent disinfection: Care in disposal of conjunctival discharges and articles soiled therewith.

   4. Terminal disinfection: None.

   5. Quarantine: None.

   6. Immunization: None.

   7. Investigation of contacts and source of infection: Examination and treatment of mother and her consort.

   8. Specific treatment: Parenteral penicillin.

   C. Epidemic measures: None; a sporadic disease.

   D. International measures: None.

GRANULOMA INGUINALE

1. *Identification.*—A mildly communicable non-fatal, chronic and progressively autoinoculable infection of skin and mucous membrane of the external genitalia, also occurring extragenitally and occasionally involving regional lymphatics. A small nodule, vesicle or papule becomes a creeping, exuberant, ulcerative, or cicatricial process of the skin, frequently painless and extending peripherally with characteristic rolled edges and formation of fibrous tissue, often with active granulomatous tissue. New lesions may occur by autoinoculation and coalesce with older ones. Local swelling may precede lesions of the inguinal region. Extragenital lesions have a predilection for warm and moist surfaces such as folds be-

tween scrotum and thighs or labia and vagina. If neglected, the disease may result in serious destruction of genital organs and spread to other parts of the body. Synonyms: Ulcerating Granuloma, Granuloma Pudenti Tropicum, Granuloma Contagiosa, Chronic Venereal Sore, and Granuloma Venereum.

Laboratory confirmation is by demonstrating the causative organism and the pathognomonic cell in stained spreads of punch biopsy tissue taken from lesions, and by histologic examination of biopsy specimens.

2. *Etiologic agent.*—Donovania granulomatis, the Donovan body.

3. *Source and reservoir of infection.*—Probably the active lesions of infected persons.

4. *Mode of transmission.*—Unknown; venereal transmission is unproved but presumably by direct contact during sexual intercourse.

5. *Incubation period.*—Unknown; presumably between 8 days and 12 weeks.

6. *Period of communicability.*—Unknown; likely during open lesions of skin or mucous membrane.

7. *Susceptibility and resistance.*—Susceptibility is variable. Immunity apparently does not follow attack.

8. *Occurrence.*—An infrequent disease of tropical, subtropical and temperate areas both north and south of the equator; apparently more frequent among males than females, and in the United States more among Negroes than whites. Predominantly at ages 20 to 40 years.

9. *Methods of control:*

A. Preventive measures:

1. Preventive measures are currently those for venereal diseases in general. See Syphilis 9A, p. 178.

B. Control of the infected individual, contacts and environment:

1. Report to local health authority: In selected endemic areas (USA, some states); not a reportable disease in most states and countries, Class 3B (p. 7).

2. Isolation: None; avoid close personal contact with others until lesions are healed.

3. Concurrent disinfection: Care in disposal of discharges from lesions and articles soiled therewith.

4. Terminal disinfection: None.

5. Quarantine: None.

6. Immunization: None.

7. Investigation of contacts and source of infection. Examination of sexual contacts with special emphasis on marital partners.

8. Specific treatment: Streptomycin, tetracycline antibiotics (aureomycin, terramycin) and chloramphenicol are effective; recurrence is to be expected in some instances, usually responding to a second course. Antimony compounds are effective but healing is slow and therapy must be continued for some months after apparent recovery.

C. Epidemic measures: Intensification of preventive and control activities.

D. International measures: See Syphilis 9D, p. 179.

HEMORRHAGIC FEVER

1. *Identification.*—An acute infectious disease characterized by fever of three to six days duration, conjunctival injection, prostration, anorexia, vomiting, hemorrhagic manifestations which begin about the third day and are an outstanding clinical feature, proteinuria about the fourth day and hypotension about the fifth; renal abnormalities continue for several weeks. About one-fourth of cases show an alarming hypotension and the majority of deaths (fatality about 6%) occur during shock. Increased fragility and permeability of capillaries are among the basic physiologic abnormalities of the disease, and contribute materially to the severe manifestations late in the first week. Convalescence is usually rapid during the third week but some loss of ability of the kidney to concentrate urine may persist for a month or so. Synonyms: Epidemic Hemorrhagic Fever, Hemorrhagic Nephroso-nephritis.

   Specific laboratory diagnostic tests are not available; clinical laboratory findings such as proteinuria, leucocytosis, thrombocytopenia and elevated nonprotein nitrogen assist in establishing the diagnosis.

   This disease is not to be confused with a number of other clinically similar acute infectious hemorrhagic fevers (Crimean, Omsk, Bukovinan and Uzbekistan) which occur in the U.S.S.R., are of viral etiology and transmitted by ticks.

2. *Etiologic agent.*—Relatively little known; Berkefeld and Seitz filtrates of infectious human materials induce hemorrhagic fever in experimentally inoculated volunteers. The agent has not been established in laboratory animals.

3. *Source and reservoir of infection.*—Assumed to be maintained in nature by a cycle involving some terrestrial arthropod and some rodent, with man only an accidental victim.

4. *Mode of transmission.*—Unknown. Epidemiologic observations in Korea suggest an analogy to scrub typhus and implicate a non-flying arthropod vector of limited mobility; trombiculid mites are a likely suggestion.

5. *Incubation period.*—Usually 12 to 16 days but varying from 9 to 35.

6. *Period of communicability.*—Not communicable from man to man.

7. *Susceptibility and resistance.*—Newcomers to endemic areas are uniformly susceptible but indigenous populations probably have some acquired resistance. Mild or inapparent infections are suspected but remain unproved in the absence of specific diagnostic tests. Second attacks have not been observed.

8. *Occurrence.*—The disease was encountered in Korea in the vicinity of the 38th parallel among United Nations troops in 1951. Earlier Russian experience in Manchuria and Siberia along the Amur River and its tributaries indicates that women and children acquire the malady, as well as men. Two seasonal outbreaks, in May and June and in October and November, account for most cases; a few occur throughout the year. The majority are isolated events but outbreaks involving 5 to 20 persons within a small unit are observed, with all infections apparently acquired at the same time and place.

9. *Methods of control:*

   A. Preventive measures: Lacking adequate information of etiologic agent and mode of transmission, preventive measures are those of diseases with an arthropod vector and a rodent host; in Korea since the summer of 1952 essentially as for Scrub Typhus (see p. 163).

B. Control of the infected individual, contacts and environment:

1. Report to local health authority: In selected endemic areas; in most countries not a reportable disease, Class 3A (p. 7).
2. Isolation: None.
3. Concurrent disinfection: None.
4. Terminal disinfection: None.
5. Quarantine: None.
6. Immunization: None.
7. Investigation of source of infection: None.
8. Specific treatment: None.

C. Epidemic measures: Since outbreaks apparently result from simultaneous infection of groups, control measures are not applicable to the episode. For measures in an endemic area, see 9A, and Scrub Typhus.

D. International measures: None.

HEPATITIS, INFECTIOUS

1. *Identification.*—An acute infection characterized by a prodromal period with constitutional manifestations, and a second phase commonly associated with jaundice and symptoms referable to liver damage. Prodromal symptoms include fever, anorexia, nausea with or without vomiting, fatigue, lassitude, headache, and abdominal discomfort. Leucopenia is usual. Fever subsides after a few days, bile may be detected in the urine, and clinically recognizable jaundice appears. The second phase is of variable duration, with occasional chronic impairment of liver function and possible cirrhosis. Convalescence may be prolonged. Severity varies greatly, from mild infection without jaundice and recognizable only by liver function test, to the rare fulminating and usually fatal acute yellow atrophy of the liver. Most infections are benign; in epidemics the fatality rarely exceeds 0.5% and commonly is nearer 0.2%. Synonyms: Epidemic Hepatitis, Epidemic Jaundice, Catarrhal Jaundice.

No specific laboratory tests are available.

2. *Etiologic agent.*—The virus of infectious hepatitis.

3. *Source and reservoir of infection.*—Feces and blood from infected persons. Presence of virus in discharges of nose and throat is poorly established; commonly assumed on epidemiological behavior of the disease.

4. *Mode of transmission.*—Probably through intimate person-to-person contact, with respiratory spread possible; transmission also occurs through transfusion of whole blood, by injection of blood serum or plasma from infected persons, and by accidental contamination of syringes or needles with traces of blood from such persons; transmissible to human volunteers by ingestion or parenteral inoculation of blood or filtered fecal suspensions from patients in the acute phase. Epidemics have been related to contaminated water, food, and milk.

5. *Incubation period.*—Long and variable, from 10 to 40 days, commonly 25 days.

6. *Period of communicability.*—Unknown; virus demonstrated in blood before clinically recognized disease; evidence of a fecal carrier state of at least 5 to 15 months. Clinical experience suggests greatest communicability from a few days before to a few days after onset, usually not exceeding 7 days.

7. *Susceptibility and resistance.*—Susceptibility is general. Degree and duration of immunity after attack unknown but probably life-long; second attacks are infrequent. No known animal other than man is susceptible.

8. *Occurrence.*—Worldwide, sporadically and in epidemics, with outbreaks most common in institutions, in rural areas, and in military forces during wars. Incidence in rural areas is decidedly higher than in cities. Most common among children and young adults, less with advancing years. Incidence highest in autumn and early winter in temperate zones.

9. *Methods of control:*

    A. Preventive measures:

        1. Good community sanitation and personal hygiene, with particular emphasis on sanitary disposal of feces and respiratory discharges.

        2. Proper technical procedure to prevent transmission by blood or blood products from an infected donor or through use of improperly sterilized syringes and needles (see Serum Hepatitis, p. 85).

    B. Control of the infected individual, contacts and environment:

        1. Report to local health authority: In selected endemic areas (USA); in most states and countries not a reportable disease, Class 3B (p. 7).

        2. Isolation: During first week of illness.

        3. Concurrent disinfection: Feces, and nose and throat secretions.

        4. Terminal disinfection: None.

        5. Quarantine: None.

        6. Immunization: Immune serum globulin, 0.01 ml. per pound of body weight intramuscularly and promptly after exposure, gives passive protection even as late as 6 days before onset of disease and lasting 6 to 8 weeks.

        7. Investigation of contacts and source of infection: Search for missed cases and surveillance of contacts.

        8. Specific treatment: None.

    C. Epidemic measures:

        1. Epidemiologic investigation to determine possible transmission by food, water, blood or blood products.

        2. Special efforts to improve sanitary and hygienic practices in the community, with the object of reducing fecal contamination of foods and water and carelessness in disposal of nose and mouth discharges.

        3. Focal concentrations of disease in schools and institutions of limited populations may suggest mass prophylaxis with immune serum globulin.

    D. International measures: None.

HEPATITIS, SERUM

1. *Identification.*—Clinically indistinguishable from infectious hepatitis (p. 83). The chief differences are a longer incubation period of serum hepatitis; that serum hepatitis is not known to be transmitted in nature from man to man; and the higher fatality varying from 6 to 12%. The relationship between the diseases is not completely understood, although the evidence suggests that each is caused by an independent virus. Synonym: Homologous Serum Jaundice.

   Absence of naturally occurring infection among associates and history of injection of blood products 2 to 6 months previously, are essential to differentiation from infectious hepatitis.

2. *Etiologic agent.*—The virus of serum hepatitis.

3. *Source and reservoir of infection.*—Blood or blood products from an infected person.

4. *Mode of transmission.*—By parenteral (intravenous, intramuscular, or subcutaneous) inoculation of infected human blood, plasma, serum or thrombin; or by administration of prophylactic or therapeutic agents with syringes and needles contaminated with traces of blood from infected persons. Immune serum globulin and albumin, although blood derivatives, do not transmit the disease.

5. *Incubation period.*—Estimated at 2 to 6 months, usually 12 to 14 weeks.

6. *Period of communicability.*—Virus is demonstrable in blood of experimentally inoculated volunteers long before symptoms. How long harbored after infection is unknown; blood donors have infected recipients in each of three successive years. Some persons are carriers without experiencing a clinically recognized attack.

7. *Susceptibility and resistance.*—Susceptibility is high, as measured by manifest disease; relatively low in children and progressively higher for adults.

8. *Occurrence.*—Worldwide in distribution, wherever appropriate circumstances exist for transmission. Incidence among recipients of pooled blood products varies from 2 to 15%, and of known icterogenic plasma as high as 60%.

9. *Methods of control:*

   A. Preventive measures:

   1. Limiting administration of whole blood, and particularly pooled blood serum or plasma, to patients or others with clear indication of therapeutic usefulness or necessity. Pooling increases the likelihood that blood products will contain the infectious agent. Use of blood substitutes free of virus, such as human albumin or dextran, where feasible. Donor recruitment programs should rigidly exclude persons with a past history of hepatitis.

   2. Thorough heat sterilization of syringes and needles, and of stylets for finger-puncture. A fresh sterile syringe and needle or stylet is essential for each patient; traces of blood from previous use contaminate these instruments.

   3. No available technical method of treatment assures destruction of serum hepatitis virus in infected blood and blood derivatives. Ultraviolet light irradiation, as now prac-

ticed, is ineffective. Recent evidence suggests storage for 6 months as a practical procedure.

B. Control of the infected individual, contacts and environment:

1. Report to local health authority: In selected endemic areas (USA) ; in most states and countries not a reportable disease, Class 3B (p. 7).

2. Isolation: None. Not known to be communicable except by injection.

3. Concurrent disinfection: Of equipment contaminated with blood.

4. Terminal disinfection: None.

5. Quarantine: None.

6. Immunization: None. Immune serum globulin of no value.

7. Investigation of contacts and source of infection: Search for groupings of cases among others who have attended in common a clinic or hospital where parenteral therapy is much employed, such as a clinic for diabetes or syphilis.

8. Specific treatment: None.

C. Epidemic measures: Surveys in areas of high incidence of persons receiving blood or blood products, to determine incidence and to control technics associated with parenteral injections.

D. International measures: None.

HERPANGINA

1. *Identification.*—An acute infection characterized by sudden onset with fever and small vesicular lesions of the pharynx which promptly ulcerate and cause moderate discomfort. The illness lasts 3 to 5 days, with occasional relapse of fever one week later ; no deaths.

Definitive diagnosis is established during acute illness by recovery of the etiologic agent from lesions, from stool specimens well into convalescence and by neutralizing and complement fixing antibody response.

Clinically, herpangina is to be distinguished from herpetic stomatitis which has larger, deeper and more painful lesions commonly located in the front of the mouth.

2. *Etiologic agent.*—At least six distinct immunologic types of Coxsackie virus, Group A.

3. *Source and reservoir of infection.*—Pharyngeal (nose and throat) discharges and feces of infected persons, frequently in the absence of clinically recognized attack.

4. *Mode of transmission.*—Direct contact with infected persons, and by droplet spread. Contaminated flies have been found, but with no reliable evidence of spread by insects, water, food or sewage.

5. *Incubation period.*—Usually 3 to 5 days.

6. *Period of communicability.*—During the acute stage of illness and perhaps longer, since the virus persists in stools for several weeks.

7. *Susceptibility and resistance.*—Susceptibility to infection is general. Immunity is acquired by infection, clinical and inapparent; duration unknown. Second attacks occur with Group A virus of different immunological type.

8. *Occurrence.*—Throughout the world, both sporadically and in epidemics, with greatest incidence in summer and early autumn. A common communicable disease of children under 10 years, but adult cases are relatively frequent.

9. *Methods of control:*

   A. Preventive measures: None.

   B. Control of the infected individual, contacts and environment:

      1. Report to local health authority: Obligatory report of epidemics; no case report, Class 4 (p. 7).

      2. Isolation: None.

      3. Concurrent disinfection: Of nose and throat discharges, feces, and articles soiled therewith.

      4. Terminal disinfection: None.

      5. Quarantine: None.

      6. Active immunization: None.

      7. Investigation of source of infection: Of no practical value.

      8. Specific treatment: None.

   C. Epidemic measures:

      1. General notice to physicians of the prevalence or increased incidence of the disease, description of usual characteristics of onset and necessity for differential diagnosis, especially from poliomyelitis.

      2. Isolation in bed of all children with fever, pending diagnosis.

   D. International measures: None.

HISTOPLASMOSIS

1. *Identification.*—Most infections are asymptomatic, with evidence of past infection limited to a positive histoplasmin skin test, and sometimes associated calcified pulmonary lesions. A generalized highly fatal form of the disease is rare, and is characterized by enlargement of the liver, spleen and lymph nodes, ulcerations of mouth, nose, pharynx and larynx, and lung lesions. Gastro-intestinal lesions are not infrequent. Recent studies of outbreaks in groups exposed in closed areas, such as a cave, storm cellar or silo, indicate that infection may result in symptoms of general malaise, weakness, fever, chest pains and nonproductive cough but with recovery the rule.

   In the rare generalized infection, the fungus is frequently seen within monocytes by microscopic examination of stained blood. Culture of blood, sternal bone marrow or exudates from ulcers confirms the diagnosis.

2. *Etiologic agent.*—Histoplasma capsulatum, a fungus.

3. *Source and reservoir of infection.*—Man is apparently infected from his environment. The fungus has been isolated from soils in areas where infection exists in man or animals; also from dogs, cats, rats, skunks, opossums and foxes.

4. *Mode of transmission.*—Presumably through inhalation of air-borne spores; possibly by ingestion of spores which contaminate food or other articles.

5. *Incubation period.*—In the few reported epidemics, symptoms appeared within 5 to 18 days after exposure.

6. *Period of communicability.*—Probably for duration of active lesions; direct transmission from man to man is unlikely.

7. *Susceptibility and resistance.*—Susceptibility is general. Inapparent infections are extremely common in endemic areas; resulting immunity is likely, but not established.

8. *Occurrence.*—Reported from widely scattered areas of North, Central and South America, Europe, Africa, Hawaii, Java and the Philippines. The disease occurs in all age groups but is more common in infants and in adults over 40 years; males outnumber females, especially at ages over ten years where the ratio is 7 to 1. Histoplasmin hypersensitivity, indicating antecedent infection, is highly prevalent in the central regions of the United States as compared with Rocky Mountain and coastal areas but with marked variation. No differences between sexes; the proportion of positive reactors increases from childhood to 30 years of age. Racial differences are not observed.

9. *Methods of control:*

A. Preventive measures: None.

B. Control of the infected individual, contacts and environment:

1. Report to local health authority: In selected endemic areas (USA); in many states and countries not a reportable disease. Reporting limited to systemic disease, Class 3B (p. 7).

2. Isolation: None.

3. Concurrent disinfection: Discharges from skin lesions and necrotic lymph nodes, sputum and articles soiled therewith.

4. Terminal disinfection: None.

5. Quarantine: None.

6. Immunization: None.

7. Investigation of contacts and source of infection: Household contacts of patients with systemic disease for evidence of infection.

8. Specific treatment: None.

C. Epidemic measures: The occurrence of grouped cases of acute pulmonary infection in an endemic area, particularly with a history of exposure to dust in a closed space, should arouse suspicion of primary histoplasmosis. Suspected places such as barns, silos, caves, and basements should be investigated.

D. International measures: None.

IMPETIGO CONTAGIOSA

1. *Identification.*—A purulent dermatitis, characterized initially by vesicular lesions which later become crusted seropurulent plaques, commonly of the face and hands, but sometimes widely over the body; a disfiguring and offensive disease but rarely serious. See page 120 for Pemphigus Neonatorum, Impetigo of the Newborn.

2. *Etiologic agent.*—Probably streptococci, with staphylococci secondarily. Crater-like ulcers of the corium commonly indicate mixed infection with hemolytic streptococcus and staphylococcus aureus.

3. *Source and reservoir of infection.*—Lesions of the skin of an infected person; possibly discharges from the nose and throat.

4. *Mode of transmission.*—By direct contact with moist discharges of skin lesions, or indirect contact with articles recently soiled by discharges. Infection may be readily inoculated from place to place on the patient's body by scratching. Some evidence of airborne transmission through dust in hospital wards for children.

5. *Incubation period.*—Usually within 5 days, often 2.

6. *Period of communicability.*—While lesions remain unhealed.

7. *Susceptibility and resistance.*—Susceptibility general, especially among children and debilitated persons.

8. *Occurrence.*—Common among children, especially in warm weather. Occurs sporadically and as small epidemics in nurseries for infants, institutions for children, and summer camps. Likely to spread rapidly where measures of personal hygiene are neglected and where other skin lesions lead to scratching; association with scabies and pediculosis is common.

9. *Methods of control:*

   A. Preventive measures:

      1. Personal cleanliness, particularly avoidance of common use of toilet articles by children.
      2. Prompt treatment of the first case in a group of children will abbreviate the period of communicability and prevent extension of lesions to new sites and to other children.
      3. Prompt treatment of parasitic infections of the skin.

   B. Control of the infected individual, contacts and environment:

      1. Report to local health authority: Obligatory report of epidemics, especially in institutions, schools, hospitals and among groups of children; no individual case report, Class 4 (p. 7).
      2. Isolation: Prevent contact with other children or debilitated persons until pustules are healed.
      3. Concurrent disinfection: Of dressings and moist discharges from the patient; sterilization of underclothes and towels before laundering; avoid reinfection from contaminated washcloths, combs, and other toilet articles.
      4. Terminal disinfection: Thorough cleaning of towels, hair brushes, combs and other toilet articles.
      5. Quarantine: None.
      6. Immunization: None.
      7. Investigation of contacts and source of infection: In family cases, of little profit; see 9C.

89

8. Specific treatment: Adequate treatment will materially shorten the period of communicability. Remove crusts with bacitracin ointment or 5% ammoniated mercury ointment; continue either with ointment or 5% ammoniated mercury in calamine lotion; 3% chlortetracycline (aureomycin) ointment is also effective. Parenteral penicillin (aqueous soluble) for severe spreading infections but never penicillin locally; chlortetracycline (aureomycin) if penicillin-resistant.

C. Epidemic measures: Child contacts should be kept under surveillance; search for skin infections among attendants of infants; persons with skin lesions should be restricted from contact with newborn babies.

D. International measures: None.

INFLUENZA

1. *Identification.*—Clinically an acute, highly communicable disease, characterized by abrupt onset with fever which lasts 1 to 6 days, chills or chilliness, aches and pains in the back and limbs, and prostration. Respiratory symptoms include coryza, sore throat and cough. Recognition is ordinarily on the basis of symptoms and the presence of an epidemic. Sporadic cases are difficult to identify. Usually a self limited disease with recovery in 48 to 72 hours; influenza derives its importance from the complications that follow, especially pneumonia in those debilitated by old age, by other disease, or in young infants.

   Laboratory confirmation is by recovery of virus from throat washings or by demonstration of a significant rise in antibodies against a specific influenza virus in serums obtained during acute and convalescent stages of the disease.

2. *Etiologic agent.*—Two types of influenza virus, Influenza A and Influenza B are long recognized; a third, Influenza C, is more recently identified. Types A and B include numerous serologically distinct strains. One strain tends to be replaced from epidemic to epidemic by another of slightly different nature; hence the importance of continued epidemiologic and serologic studies.

3. *Source and reservoir of infection.*—Discharges from the mouth and nose of infected persons.

4. *Mode of transmission.*—By direct contact, through droplet infection, or by articles freshly soiled with discharges of the nose and throat of infected persons; possibly air-borne.

5. *Incubation period.*—Short, usually 24 to 72 hours.

6. *Period of communicability.*—Probably limited to one week after onset.

7. *Susceptibility and resistance.*—Susceptibility is close to universal but of varying degree, as evidenced by frequent inapparent and atypical infections during epidemics. After early infancy, presence of serum antibody is a result of infection. For a population, antibody content for different types of virus, and varieties within types is a reflection of the experience of that population; for individuals it tends to broaden with age and to exist in varying degree and ex-

tent. Immunity after attack may persist for several years against homologous or closely related strains, but freedom from disease is often short because of the variety of influenza viruses and of other microbial agents capable of inducing the influenzal syndrome.

8. *Occurrence.*—Variable, in pandemics, local epidemics and as sporadic cases, the latter commonly unrecognized. Epidemics may affect up to half a population within 4 to 6 weeks; attack rates ordinarily vary from less than 5 to 20 to 30%. The latest highly fatal pandemic of influenza, representing a worldwide distribution of the infectious agent, occurred in 1918; those since then have been milder and less widespread. In temperate zones epidemics tend to occur in winter, in the tropics irregularly. The disease shows a cyclic tendency, with influenza A appearing in epidemic form at shorter intervals than does influenza B. A single serologic type of virus is usually present among patients of the same epidemic, but presence of two types is known.

9. *Methods of control:*

    A. Preventive measures:

        1. Education of the public as to sanitary hazards from spitting, sneezing and coughing in the close presence of other persons with stress that the viruses of influenza are in discharges from the upper respiratory tract. Avoid use of common towels, glasses, eating utensils, or toilet articles and encourage use of disposable paper handkerchiefs and napkins.

        2. Active immunization with currently available vaccines achieves a substantial reduction in incidence of influenza, provided the prevailing strain of virus matches closely the antigenic components of the vaccine used. Opinion differs on duration of protection but immunization oftener than once a year appears unnecessary. Major shifts in antigenic structure of influenza virus occur and discount the effectiveness of general immunization programs.

        Inoculation with vaccine during an epidemic is valueless; the disease spreads rapidly and protection does not follow until seven days. For practical effect, must be employed in advance of an anticipated epidemic; international control measures under D2 and D3 below are designed to make this possible. The same procedures are applicable within a country.

        General inoculation of whole populations is not feasible, but experimental use of influenza vaccines under controlled conditions is increasingly practiced for selected groups.

    B. Control of the infected individual, contacts and environment:

        1. Report to local health authority: Obligatory report of epidemics resembling influenza; no individual case report, Class 4 (p. 7). Confirmation of the epidemic disease as influenza should be sought promptly through laboratory procedures.

        2. Isolation: During the acute illness; not as an official requirement but as directed by the attending physician.

        3. Concurrent disinfection: Discharges from the nose and throat of the patient.

4. Terminal disinfection: None.
5. Quarantine: None.
6. Immunization: Of contacts, none.
7. Investigation of contacts and source of infection: Of no practical value.
8. Specific treatment: None. Sulfonamides and antibiotics do not affect the uncomplicated disease; should be employed if pulmonary complications arise.

C. Epidemic measures:

1. To minimize severity and to protect the patient from secondary infections thus reducing mortality, patients should go to bed at the beginning of an attack and not return to work without the approval of a physician.
2. The aggregation of large numbers of persons is to be discouraged. The closing of schools is not effective in checking spread.
3. Crowding of beds in hospitals and institutions to accommodate increased numbers of patients and other inmates is especially to be avoided. Increased spacing between beds in wards and dormitories reduces risk of attack and of pneumonia.
4. Continued dissemination of current information on extent and nature of the epidemic to local health authorities by state or national health agencies.

D. International measures:

1. Prompt notification to WHO of epidemics within a country, especially those involving institutional, military or other considerable groups.
2. Identification of virus type in such situations through prompt dispatch of the necessary blood samples or throat washings to one of the official influenza virus detection centers which now number close to 60, and are widely distributed in many countries. The World Influenza Center is in London.
3. Continuing epidemiologic studies and exchange of information by official health agencies in order to establish broad movements of epidemic influenza, to facilitate early recognition of outbreaks within a country, and to identify the prevailing type and strain of virus.

KERATOCONJUNCTIVITIS

1. *Identification.*—An acute infection of the eye, characterized by fever, headache, edema of lids, scleral injection, follicular hypertrophy of palpebral conjunctiva, enlargement and tenderness of preauricular lymph nodes and a watery conjunctival discharge, sometimes followed by multiple pinpoint corneal opacities which usually heal readily but may persist indefinitely. Involvement usually bilateral. The onset is commonly acute, with sensation of a foreign body under the upper lid. Ocular sequelae are unusual and the disease is non-fatal. Synonyms: Infectious Punctate Keratitis, Nummular Keratitis.

Confirmation of clinical diagnosis is by smears of conjunctival scrapings showing mononuclear cells and by absence of etiologic agents of other forms of conjunctivitis.

2. *Etiologic agent.*—Unknown; probably due to one or more viruses.

3. *Source and reservoir of infection.*—Probably the discharge from the eye of an infected person or a carrier.

4. *Mode of transmission.*—Apparently through direct contact with an infected person or with articles freshly soiled with conjunctival and nasal discharges of such person. Spread of infection by hands and instruments during the course of ophthalmic examination has been reported.

5. *Incubation period.*—Not definitely established, but probably about 5 to 7 days.

6. *Period of communicability.*—Unknown but certainly during acute stage of the disease.

7. *Susceptibility and resistance.*—Susceptibility variable. No age, sex or race is known to be immune.

8. *Occurrence.*—In epidemics in warm climates, also among industrial employees in temperate climates and involving only a small proportion of groups affected.

9. *Methods of control:*

   A. Preventive measures:

      1. Education as to personal cleanliness and as to danger of use of common towels and toilet articles.
      2. Avoid contamination of hands with conjunctival or nasal discharges.
      3. Aseptic technic in professional care of patients with eye diseases and injuries.

   B. Control of the infected individual, contacts and environment:

      1. Report to local health authority: Obligatory report of epidemic; no individual case report, Class 4 (p. 7).
      2. Isolation: None; hygienic measures by the infected person.
      3. Concurrent disinfection: Of conjunctival and nasal discharges and articles soiled therewith.
      4. Terminal disinfection: None.
      5. Quarantine: None.
      6. Immunization: None.
      7. Investigation of contacts and source of infection: To locate other cases and institute precautions at home or working place.
      8. Specific treatment: None; appropriate antibiotics for the control of secondary infection.

   C. Epidemic measures:

      1. Intensify educational efforts with respect to eye hygiene.
      2. Organize convenient facilities for prompt diagnosis and treatment of patients.

   D. International measures: None.

LEISHMANIASIS, CUTANEOUS

1. *Identification.*—Localized superficial infection of reticuloendothelial macrophages by Leishmania, producing nodular and ulcerating indolent lesions of any exposed part of the body. Each lesion is the result of a bite by an individual infected insect vector, except for secondary lesions produced by scratching. In some parts of tropical America and Africa the lesions are more ulcerative, and often involve mucous membranes, causing extensive necrosis of nose, mouth and pharynx; secondary infection and complications may cause death. Synonyms: In Old World: Oriental Sore, Aleppo, Baghdad or Delhi Boil; in New World: Espundia, Uta, Chiclero Ulcer.

   Definitive diagnosis is by microscopic identification of Leishmania bodies in scrapings from edges of lesions, smeared on a glass slide and stained as for a blood smear; also by culture on suitable media of material aspirated from lesions.

2. *Etiologic agent.*—Leishmania tropica (old world). Leishmania braziliensis (new world).

3. *Source and reservoir of infection.*—Sandflies are the immediate source; persons with exposed lesions containing parasites are reservoirs of infection, also dogs, cats and Turkestan gerbils.

4. *Mode of transmission.*—Commonly through bite of infected sandflies of the genus Phlebotomus; perhaps mechanically by other flies or by direct contact of abraded skin with lesion of another person, but doubtful.

5. *Incubation period.*—From a few weeks to many months.

6. *Period of communicability.*—As long as parasites remain in lesions. In untreated cases this may be for a year or longer. Spontaneous healing is the rule except in cases with destructive mucous membrane involvement. Duration of infectivity of vector unknown.

7. *Susceptibility and resistance.*—Susceptibility is general. A healed lesion is associated with immunity.

8. *Occurrence.*—Old World: northwest India, west Pakistan, the Middle East, southern Russia, the Mediterranean littoral, north, west and central Africa. New World: endemic in Mexico (especially Yucatan), most of Central America, and every country of South America except Chile. Occasionally seen in the United States in persons coming from endemic areas.

9. *Methods of control:*

   A. Preventive measures:

      1. Periodic application of insecticide having residual action to exterior and interior of doorways and all other openings in habitations through which Phlebotomus can enter. This insect flies in small "hops," spends much time on surfaces, and thus is especially vulnerable to contact insecticides. Possible breeding places should be sprayed in rubbish, stone walls, duck and chicken pens, animal houses and similar damp situations near dwellings.

      2. Residual spraying may be supplemented by aerosol spraying of bed nets, and use of insect repellents.

94

3. Sanitary housing, providing adequate light and ventilation, and eliminating damp floors, thatched roofs, rubbish, vegetation near house, and animals stabled in the house.

4. Vaccination using scrapings from active lesions of oriental sore has been practiced successfully by native peoples. Active immunization with a live vaccine of L. tropica prepared from cultures or infected developing chick embryo, provides protection against oriental sore. No immunizing procedure against L. braziliensis.

5. Education of the population concerning the mode of transmission and methods of controlling Phlebotomus.

B. Control of the infected individual, contacts and environment:

1. Report to local health authority: In selected endemic areas; in many countries not a reportable disease, Class 3B (p. 7).

2. Isolation: None; protect patient from bites of Phlebotomus by fine mesh screens and mosquito nets (45 to the linear inch), by spraying of quarters with insecticide having residual action and by the use of repellents.

3. Concurrent disinfection: None, other than destruction of sandflies in dwelling.

4. Terminal disinfection: None, other than destruction of sandflies in dwelling.

5. Quarantine: None.

6. Immunization: Active immunization, for L. tropica infection, oriental sore.

7. Investigation of contacts and source of infection: Search for other cases among contacts and for Phlebotomus; also breeding areas of sandflies around dwellings.

8. Specific treatment: Neostibosan as for kala azar. Recovery may be expected within four weeks. Secondary bacterial infection is treated with appropriate systemic or local antibiotic or by chemotherapy.

C. Epidemic measures: In areas of high incidence intensive efforts to control the disease by provision of diagnostic facilities, by mass treatment campaigns and by anti-phlebotomus measures.

D. International measures: None.

LEISHMANIASIS, VISCERAL

1. *Identification.*—A protozoan infection of the reticuloendothelial system, characterized by fever, splenomegaly, hepatomegaly, lymphadenopathy, leucopenia, and progressive emaciation and weakness. Untreated cases nearly always end fatally. Fever is of gradual or sudden onset, often with two daily peaks; alternating periods of apyrexia and low grade fever follow. Common complications are pneumonia, gangrenous stomatitis, dysentery. After chemotherapy cutaneous lesions containing Leishmania may occur. Synonym: Kala Azar.

Diagnosis is by finding Leishman-Donovan bodies in stained smears from bone marrow, spleen, liver or lymph node puncture, rarely and late in blood smears; by culture of such materials, or injection into hamsters. Globulin precipitation and complement fixation are presumptive tests.

2. *Etiologic agent.*—Leishmania donovani (L. infantum).

3. *Source and reservoir of infection.*—Immediate source is Phlebotomus; reservoir is usually man, in reticuloendothelial cells or blood in advanced stages. The high incidence of the infection among dogs and cats in some endemic areas suggests these animals as reservoirs of human infection.

4. *Mode of transmission.*—Through bite of infected sandflies of the genus Phlebotomus. The fly is infected by sucking the perpiheral blood or by ingesting parasites present in skin of an infected individual.

5. *Incubation period.*—Generally 2 to 4 months; as short as 10 days or as long as 19 months.

6. *Period of communicability.*—As long as the parasites persist in circulating blood or in skin, occasionally after treatment and clinical recovery from visceral infection. Duration of infectivity of sandfly is unknown.

7. *Susceptibility and resistance.*—Susceptibility is general. In the Mediterranean area most cases occur in children under 5 years of age. In other endemic areas the peak of incidence is 5 to 15 years, with many cases in adults. Clinical recovery apparently leads to lasting immunity.

8. *Occurrence.*—Endemic in China, chiefly north of the Yangtse as far as south Manchuria; east Pakistan and India (Bengal, Assam and Madras); Mediterranean basin (Italy, Greece, Malta, Corsica, Aegean Islands, Jordan, Palestine, South Spain, Turkey); also Portugal, Jugoslavia, Hungary; Transcaucasia, Russian Turkestan; North Africa (Morocco, Tunis, Algeria); some areas in tropical Africa (Sudan, Ethiopia, northern Kenya); South America (Argentina and Brazil).

9. *Methods of control:*

   A. Preventive measures:

      1. Periodic application of insecticide having residual action to exterior and interior of doorways and all other openings in habitations through which Phlebotomus can enter. This insect flies in small "hops" and thus is especially vulnerable to contact insecticides. Phlebotomus control may be incidental to adult mosquito control for malaria. Possible breeding places in rubbish, stone walls, and other situations near dwellings should be sprayed.

      2. Residual spraying may be supplemented by aerosol spraying of bed nets, and use of insect repellents.

      3. Sanitary housing, providing adequate light and ventilation, and eliminating damp floors, thatched roofs, rubbish, vegetation near houses, and animals stabled in the house.

      4. Provision of diagnostic and large-scale treatment campaigns reduces opportunity for infection of sandflies.

      5. Destruction of all stray and infected dogs in regions of high human endemicity.

      6. Education of the population concerning mode of transmission and methods of Phlebotomus control.

B. Control of the infected individual, contacts and environment:

1. Report to local health authority: In selected endemic areas; in many countries not a reportable disease, Class 3B (p. 7).

2. Isolation: None. Protect patient from bites of Phlebotomus by fine mesh screens and mosquito nets, by spraying quarters with insecticide having residual action, and by use of repellents.

3. Concurrent disinfection: None.

4. Terminal disinfection: None.

5. Quarantine: None.

6. Immunization: None.

7. Investigation of contacts and source of infection: Search for sandflies on the immediate premises or for other contact with them.

8. Specific treatment: Neostibosan intravenously; where the infectious agent is resistant to antimony therapy (in the Egyptian Sudan), the diamidine compounds (Stilbamidine, Pentamidine) may be effective; side effects require caution. In the Mediterranean area the parasite is more resistant than in India and requires more energetic treatment.

C. Epidemic measures:

1. Surveys in areas of high incidence and location of endemic foci.

2. Intensive efforts to eliminate the disease by mass treatment campaigns and by anti-phlebotomus measures.

D. International measures: Coordinated programs of control entered into by neighboring countries where the disease is endemic.

LEPROSY

1. *Identification.*—A chronic communicable disease characterized by lesions of the skin—infiltration, macules, plaques, papules and nodules—and by involvement of peripheral nerves with consequent anesthesia, muscle weakness and paralysis, and trophic changes in skin, muscle and bone. In lepromatous (cutaneous) leprosy, the mucous membranes of the upper respiratory tract are also usually invaded. Progress of the disease is slow but ultimate fatality is high.

Demonstration of acid-fast bacilli in suspected lesions is confirmatory in lepromatous cases; bacilli may be rare or not demonstrable in tuberculoid (maculo-anesthetic) lesions and diagnosis depends primarily upon presence of anesthesia in areas served by affected nerves.

2. *Etiologic agent.*—Mycobacterium leprae, leprosy bacillus.

3. *Source and reservoir of infection.*—Discharges from lesions of infected persons.

4. *Mode of transmission.*—Not definitely known; the bacillus probably gains entrance through skin or mucous membrane of the upper respiratory tract.

5. *Incubation period.*—Prolonged, undetermined, from one to several years.

6. *Period of communicability.*—Commences when lesions become open and discharge leprosy bacilli; continues until healing, communicability being shortened by adequate chemotherapy. Patients with demonstrable acid-fast bacilli in smears from skin or mucous membrane are potentially open cases even if demonstrable ulceration is not present.

7. *Susceptibility and resistance.*—No racial immunity. More frequent in persons exposed in early life; the lesser incidence among adults is seemingly dependent on differences in opportunity for infection.

8. *Occurrence.*—Mostly in the tropics and subtropics. Prevalence rates of 5 per 1,000 or higher are found only in the tropics. A few countries with temperate climates have estimated rates of 1 : 1,000, including China, Japan and Korea. China and India have about one-half of the estimated world total of 3 to 4 million cases. In Europe, low endemicity in Greece, Portugal, Spain; residual foci only in several other countries. Endemic but decreasing in Hawaii, present at a low level in Canal Zone, Puerto Rico and Virgin Islands, and in continental United States, chiefly limited to Gulf Coast areas of Florida, Louisiana and Texas.

9. *Methods of control:*

  A. Preventive measures:

    1. In endemic areas leprosy is usually contracted in childhood but may be acquired in adult life. Infants should be separated from leprous parents at birth; educational efforts should stress greater risk when exposure is early in life. The exaggerated fear of leprosy and belief in its high communicability should be discounted.

  B. Control of the infected individual, contacts and environment:

    1. Report to local health authority: Case report obligatory in most states and countries and desirable in all, Class 2B (p. 7).

    2. Isolation: In endemic areas, patients with demonstrable leprosy bacilli in smears from the lesions should be isolated in hospitals or colonies and treated until bacteriologically negative for at least six months. The next best procedure is institutional treatment until ulcerative lesions are healed followed by home isolation with medical supervision. In many countries of high endemicity only clinic supervision is practicable. In areas where the disease is not indigenous, home isolation is sufficient. Patients discharged from institutions should be examined periodically, the suggested interval being six months.

    3. Concurrent disinfection: Discharges of lesions and articles soiled therewith.

    4. Terminal disinfection: Thorough cleaning of living premises of patient.

    5. Quarantine: None.

    6. Immunization: None.

    7. Investigation of contacts and source of infection: Should be undertaken in cases of apparently recent origin; the long and uncertain period of incubation makes discovery of

the source of infection difficult. Periodic examination of contacts for secondary cases.

8. Specific treatment: Sulfones (promin, diasone and D.D.S., di-amino-diphenyl sulfone), the preferred therapeutic agents, are continued for long periods. Promin is administered intravenously, diasone orally, with slowly increased doses. Initial small oral doses of D.D.S. are slowly increased to tolerance. Streptomycin probably has value equal to sulfones and may be substituted when sulfone therapy fails or is not tolerated. Isoniazid and a number of other drugs are under evaluation. Penicillin is of value only for control of secondary infection.

C. Epidemic measures: In areas giving evidence of spread of infection (high endemicity or those uncommon situations justifying epidemic characterization) provision of facilities for bacteriological diagnosis, treatment clinics, case finding to include examination of family contacts of known cases every six months, separation of children of leprous parents from birth and repatriation of immigrants developing the disease within five years of arrival; also the usual measures of reporting and isolation.

D. International measures:

1. Exercise of the recognized international rights of governments to refuse entry of immigrants who are found to have leprosy is usual and desirable.

2. Reciprocal measures between governments at authorized points of entry of immigrants to prevent introduction or spread of the disease.

LEPTOSPIROSIS

1. *Identification.*—An acute systemic infection characterized by fever, chills, severe malaise and muscular aches, headache, vomiting, stiff neck, injection of conjunctivae, and infrequently jaundice, renal insufficiency, hemolytic anemia, and hemorrhage in skin and mucous membranes. Leucocytosis is common, pleocytosis of spinal fluid frequent. The acute illness lasts from one to three weeks; relapses may occur. Case fatality is low; in severe cases with jaundice and kidney damage, formerly considered the common manifestations of the disease, may reach 20% or more, being greater with advancing age. Synonyms: Weil's Disease, Canicola Fever, Swineherd Disease, Mud Fever, Hemorrhagic Jaundice.

2. *Etiologic agent.*—Many species of the genus Leptospira; L. icterohemorrhagiae, L. canicola and a member of the sero-group autumnalis have been recovered from human cases in the United States; and in addition serologic evidence of human infection with members of the serogroup pomona, bataviae and grippotyphosa; others are probable. At present at least 21 serogroups containing 35 serotypes are recognized.

3. *Source and reservoir of infection.*—The source is urine of chronically infected animals and possibly infected tissues. Reservoirs include cattle, dogs and swine, rats and other wild rodents.

4. *Mode of transmission.*—Contact with water contaminated with urine of infected animals, as in swimming or accidental immersion; direct contact with infected animals. Infection presumably results from penetration of abraded skin or mucous membrane, or possibly from ingestion.

5. *Incubation period.*—Four to 19 days, usually 10 days.

6. *Period of communicability.*—Communicability from man to man is negligible.

7. *Susceptibility and resistance.*—Susceptibility of man is general. Demonstrable antibodies are generally present in serum up to one year; may persist for many years.

8. *Occurrence.*—Outbreaks among swimmers exposed to contaminated waters are reported with increasing frequency. An occupational hazard to veterinarians, animal husbandmen, abattoir workers, fish workers, and those who live or work in rat-infested premises. Distribution of reservoirs of infection and of one or another species of leptospira is probably world wide.

9. *Methods of control:*

A. Preventive measures:
1. Protection with boots and gloves of workers exposed to hazard of infection.
2. Avoidance of swimming in potentially contaminated waters.
3. Rodent control in human habitations, particularly rural and recreational.
4. Segregation of domestic animals and prevention of contamination of human living and working areas by urine of infected animals.

B. Control of the infected individual, contacts and environment:
1. Report to local health authority: Obligatory case report in many states and countries, Class 2B (p. 7).
2. Isolation: None.
3. Concurrent disinfection: None.
4. Terminal disinfection: None.
5. Quarantine: None.
6. Immunization: None of established value.
7. Investigation of contacts and source of infection: Search for exposure to infected animals or swimming in contaminated waters.
8. Specific treatment: Penicillin, streptomycin, and the tetracycline antibiotics are leptospirocidal in vitro, but not yet of demonstrated value in treatment of human infections.

C. Epidemic measures: Search for source of infection, such as a swimming pool; eliminate contamination, or prohibit further use.

D. International measures: None.

LYMPHOCYTIC CHORIOMENINGITIS

1. *Identification.*—An endemic viral infection of animals, especially mice, transmissible to man with a marked diversity of clinical manifestations; may begin with an influenza-like attack and terminate by recovery, or after a few days of more or less complete remission, meningeal symptoms suddenly appear. Attack is sometimes initiated by meningeal symptoms. Severe meningoencephalitic cases have somnolence, disturbed deep reflexes, paralysis, and anaesthesia of skin. Course is usually short and most patients recover within a few weeks; occasionally fatal. Spinal fluid, sterile to bacterial culture, has from a few hundred to more than 3,500 cells per cmm., almost wholly lymphocytes.

   Laboratory diagnostic methods include isolation of virus from blood, urine, nasopharynx or spinal fluid early in attack; inoculation of guinea pigs intraperitoneally or of mice intracerebrally; or comparison of titers of neutralizing or complement fixing antibodies in serums collected early and late in the disease, an interval of 6 weeks often being necessary.

   Other causes of sterile meningitis require differentiation, including leptospirosis, mumps, poliomyelitis and other encephalitides.

2. *Etiologic agent.*—The virus of lymphocytic choriomeningitis.

3. *Source and reservoir of infection.*—The infected house mouse, Mus musculus musculus. Naturally infected guinea pigs, monkeys, dogs and swine have been observed.

4. *Mode of transmission.*—The virus escapes from infected animals in mouth and nasal secretions, urine, and feces. Transmission to man is probably through contaminated food or dust, possibly by arthropods.

5. *Incubation period.*—Information is limited; probably 8 to 13 days from infection to systemic manifestations, 15 to 21 days to meningeal symptoms.

6. *Period of communicability.*—Not communicable in nature from man to man. Naturally infected mice may carry the virus through life; the infected female transmits virus to offspring.

7. *Susceptibility and resistance.*—Unknown; virus neutralization by blood serum of persons recovered from the disease and of many without history of recognized attack is commonly observed.

8. *Occurrence.*—Rare, but more common than the number of recognized cases indicates. Foci of infection often persist within limits of a city block for months or years, giving sporadic clinical disease.

9. *Methods of control:*

   A. Preventive measures:

      1. General cleanliness of home and place of work, with elimination of mice.

   B. Control of the infected individual, contacts, and environment:

      1. Report to local health authority: Official report not ordinarily justifiable, Class 5 (p. 7).

      2. Isolation: None.

      3. Concurrent disinfection: Of discharges from the nose and throat, of urine and feces, and of articles soiled therewith.

    4. Terminal disinfection: None.

    5. Quarantine: None.

    6. Immunization: None.

    7. Investigation of contacts and source of infection: Home and place of employment for presence of house mice with attention also to arthropods.

    8. Specific treatment: None.

C. Epidemic measures: Not applicable.

D. International measures: None.

LYMPHOGRANULOMA VENEREUM

1. *Identification.*—A venereally acquired virus infection of lymph channels and lymph nodes manifesting itself in a variety of ways: bubo formations, ulcerations, elephantiasis of genitalia, and rectal stricture. The disease sometimes begins with a small painless evanescent erosion, papule, or herpetiform lesion, followed shortly by acute, subacute or chronic adenitis and periadenitis, usually with multiple foci of suppuration and with grooved adherent skin of a purplish hue; more commonly the bubo is the first manifestation. Constitutional symptoms during lymphatic progression include fever, chills, headache, vague abdominal aches, joint pains and anorexia. Spontaneous regression of buboes does not indicate recovery; the course is often long, disability is great, but the disease is essentially nonfatal. Synonyms: Lymphogranuloma Inguinale, Climatic Bubo, Poradenitis, and Lymphopathia Venereum.

    Diagnosis is aided by skin test with Frei antigen or by demonstration of complement fixing antibodies against lymphogranuloma venereum-psittacosis group of viruses; neither test is conclusive.

2. *Etiologic agent.*—The virus of lymphogranuloma venereum, immunologically related to virus of psittacosis.

3. *Source and reservoir of infection.*—Lesions of rectum and urethra and sinuses and ulcerations of infected persons.

4. *Mode of transmission.*—Through direct contact during sexual intercourse; by indirect contact with articles contaminated by infectious exudates, especially infections acquired by children.

5. *Incubation period.*—5 to 21 days to primary lesion, usually 7 to 12; if inguinal bubo is first manifestation, 10 to 30 days, sometimes several months.

6. *Period of communicability.*—Variable, from weeks to years, during presence of active lesions.

7. *Susceptibility and resistance.*—Susceptibility seemingly is general. Immunity does not follow attack; no artificial immunity.

8. *Occurrence.*—A commoner disease than ordinarily believed; widespread throughout the world, especially tropical and subtropical areas. Endemic in southern United States, particularly among Negroes. Age incidence is that of greatest sexual activity, with the disease most frequent among the sexually promiscuous. Sex differences are not pronounced and all races are affected.

9. *Methods of control:*

A. Preventive measures:

1. Except for specific information relating to lymphogranuloma venereum, preventive measures are those for the venereal diseases (see Syphilis 9A, p. 178).

B. Control of the infected individual, contacts and environment:

1. Report to local health authority: In selected endemic areas (USA some states); in most states and countries not a reportable disease, Class 3C (p. 7).

2. Isolation: Avoid sexual contact until lesions are healed.

3. Concurrent disinfection: None; care in disposal of discharges from lesions and of articles soiled therewith.

4. Terminal disinfection: None.

5. Quarantine: None.

6. Immunization: None.

7. Investigation of contacts and source of infection: Search for sexual contacts exposed prior and subsequent to appearance of disease.

8. Specific treatment: Varies with stage; chlortetracycline (aureomycin) in the bubo phase, with sulfadiazine moderately successful; for proctitis and other ulcerative lesions, tetracycline antibiotics (aureomycin, terramycin), chloramphenicol or sulfadiazine, administered for 30 days or more after discharges subside.

C. Epidemic measures: Intensification of preventive and control activities.

D. International measures: See Syphilis 9D, p. 179.

MALARIA

1. *Identification.*—A severe systemic disease, acute and often chronic, commonly beginning with a brief and indefinite illness shortly followed by a characteristic shaking chill with rapidly rising temperature, usually accompanied by headache and nausea and ending with profuse sweating; after an interval free of fever, the cycle of chills, fever and sweating is repeated. As the disease progresses the paroxysms tend to occur daily, every other day or every third day, depending on the species of the etiologic agent. The duration of untreated primary attack varies from a week to a month or longer. Relapses are common and may occur at irregular intervals for several years. Fatality in untreated cases varies from less than 1% to 10% or even higher, depending on character of the parasite and degree of host resistance. In treated cases the rate may be 0.1% and rarely exceeds 0.5%. Clinical diagnosis depends upon development of the characteristic recurrent chills and fever, enlargement of the spleen and secondary anemia, often with palpable spleen and mild icterus.

Laboratory confirmation should always be sought through demonstration of malaria parasites in blood films by microscopic examination. Repeated examinations may be necessary; the thick film method is most likely to reveal the parasite; often not demonstrable in films from patients recently or actively under treatment.

2. *Etiologic agent.*—Plasmodium vivax for tertian malaria, P. malariae for quartan malaria, P. falciparum for falciparum malaria and P. ovale for the rare ovale malaria.

3. *Source and reservoir of infection.*—The immediate source is an infected mosquito. Man is the only known reservoir.

4. *Mode of transmission.*—Certain species of Anopheles ingest human blood containing plasmodia in the gametocyte stage and act as definitive hosts. The parasite develops into sporozoites in from 8 to 35 days depending on species of parasite and temperature to which the insect is exposed. Sporozoites lodge in the salivary glands and are injected into man as the insect thereafter takes a blood meal. In the susceptible host, gametocytes usually appear in the blood within 3 to 14 days, according to species of parasite. Malaria may be transmitted also by injection or transfusion of blood of infected persons or by use of contaminated hypodermic syringes, as by drug addicts.

5. *Incubation period.*—Average 12 days for P. falciparum, 13 to 15 days for P. vivax, and 28 to 30 days for P. malariae. With some strains of P. vivax, primary attack may be delayed for 8 to 10 months, the period of latency being known as protracted incubation period. With infection by blood transfusion, incubation may be much shorter.

6. *Period of communicability.*—As long as infective gametocytes circulate in the blood; varies with species and strain of parasite and with response to therapy. May extend indefinitely in quartan malaria, from 1 to 3 years in vivax, and rarely more than 1 year in falciparum. The infected mosquito remains infective for long periods; only the female takes blood meals.

7. *Susceptibility and resistance.*—Susceptibility is universal; the degree of susceptibility is sometimes lessened by previous infection. A high degree of tolerance to the effects of infection may develop in highly endemic primitive communities where exposure to infective anophelines is continuous over many years.

8. *Occurrence.*—Highly infrequent in the United States and in several other countries where malaria was a health problem a decade ago. A number of countries in the tropics, with a tradition of hyperendemic malaria, have now greatly reduced the incidence by modern control measures. The disease is still a major cause of ill health in many parts of tropical and subtropical Africa, Asia, and the Southwest Pacific.

9. *Methods of control:*

   A. Preventive measures:

      1. Application of residual insecticide (such as DDT, benzene hexachloride or dieldrin) in suitable formula and dosage at appropriate intervals on the inside walls of dwellings and on other surfaces upon which vector anophelines habitually rest will generally result in effective malaria control. Usually entire communities are included in a spraying project and the latter is routinely carried forward year after year until malaria ceases to be endemic.

      2. Where residual insecticide is not available, nightly spraying of living and sleeping quarters with a liquid or an aerosol preparation of pyrethrum is useful.

3. In endemic areas, living and sleeping quarters should be screened and bed nets used.

4. Insect repellents (such as dimethylphthalate or 2-ethylhexane-diol, 1, 3, commonly called "612") applied to uncovered skin and impregnated in the clothing of persons exposed to bites of vector anophelines are useful.

5. Sanitary improvements, such as filling and draining, to eliminate breeding places of vector anophelines should not be neglected. Larvicides (such as oil and Paris green) are now not commonly used where residual spraying is effective but may have usefulness under special conditions.

6. Regular use of suppressive drugs in highly malarious areas has special value (see 9B8).

7. Effective treatment of acute and chronic cases is an important adjunct to malaria control.

8. Malaria control projects often profit from health education that teaches modern drug treatment and suppression, and practical measures of prevention.

B. Control of the infected individual, contacts and environment:

1. Report to local health authority: Obligatory case report, Class 2B (p. 7), in non-endemic areas and in areas where the disease has been brought under control, desirably limited to authenticated cases (USA). Class 3C (p. 7) is the more practical procedure in endemic areas.

2. Isolation: None; patients desirably are protected at night by screens or bed nets in areas where vector anophelines are present.

3. Concurrent disinfection: A single concurrent residual spraying of the neighborhood may be useful, if a primary or relapsing case occurs in an area not under control, previously free from the disease and where potential vectors are active.

4. Terminal disinfection: None.

5. Quarantine: None.

6. Immunization: None.

7. Investigation of contacts and source of infection: Determine history of previous infection or of exposure to infection by anophelines or otherwise.

8. Specific treatment: (a) Acute cases in non-immune subjects: Chloroquine diphosphate or sulphate 600 mgm. (base) immediately, followed in six hours by 300 mgm. (base), and 300 mgm. (base) on each of next two days; or amodiaquine dihydrochloride dihydrate, same regimen and dosage as above. (b) Acute cases, emergency treatment: Mepacrine methane sulphonate 400 mgm. intramuscularly, repeated after six hours if necessary; or chloroquine hydrochloride, 200 or 300 mgm. intramuscularly, repeated after 6 hours if the patient is not able to take additional drug (i.e. diphosphate) by mouth; or quinine hydrobromide or dihydrochloride 600 mgm. well diluted in normal saline, administered intravenously and slowly, and repeated after six hours if necessary. (c) Acute cases in semi-immune subjects: Chloroquine diphosphate or sulphate in a single dose 600 mgm. (base); or amo-

diaquine dihydrochloride dihydrate, in a single dose 600 mgm. (base).

Suppression: Chloroquine diphosphate or sulphate, 300 mgm. (base) once weekly preferably on the same day each week; or amodiaquine dihydrochloride dihydrate, 300 or 400 mgm. (base) once weekly; or proguanil mono-hydrochloride, 100 mgm. daily, or for semi-immune subjects, 300 mgm. once weekly; or pyrimethamine, 25 mgm. once weekly.

Prevention of relapse: Primaquine diphosphate, 15 mgm. (base) daily for 14 days; should be given to persons leaving endemic areas at time suppressive drugs are discontinued. In acute attacks, may be given concurrently with standard chloroquine or amodiaquine treatment.

C. Epidemic measures: A field survey to determine nature and extent of the hyperendemic or epidemic situation is the point of departure. Intensify residual spraying, treatment of acute cases, and use of suppressive drugs. Sometimes the breeding places of anophelines responsible for an epidemic can be eliminated.

D. International measures:

1. Routine disinsectization of aircraft coming from malarial areas. Special disinsectization of aircraft, ships and other vehicles not possessing a valid disinsectization certificate, prior to arrival in areas freed from anophelines generally or from certain species.

2. So far as practicable, rigid anti-mosquito sanitation should be maintained within the mosquito flight range of all ports and airports.

MEASLES

1. *Identification.*—An acute highly communicable viral disease with a prodromal stage characterized by catarrhal symptoms and Koplik spots on the buccal mucous membranes. A morbilliform rash appears on the third or fourth day affecting face, body and extremities, and sometimes ending in branny desquamation. Leucopenia is usual. Death from uncomplicated measles is rare. Such deaths as occur are usually the result of secondary pneumonia, in children under 2 years old and the aggregate is less than 1 per 1,000 cases of measles. Synonyms: Rubeola, Morbilli.

Virus isolation and serological identification of measles are not practicable.

2. *Etiologic agent.*—The virus of measles.

3. *Source and reservoir of infection.*—Secretions of nose and throat of infected persons.

4. *Mode of transmission.*—By droplet spread or direct contact with an infected person; indirectly through articles freshly soiled with secretions of nose and throat. One of the most readily transmitted of communicable diseases; in some instances probably airborne.

5. *Incubation period.*—About 10 days from exposure to initial fever; about 14 days until rash appears; uncommonly longer or shorter. Late inoculation in attempted passive protection may extend incubation to 21 days.

6. *Period of communicability.*—During the period of catarrhal symptoms; usually about 9 days, from 4 days before to 5 days after rash appears.

7. *Susceptibility and resistance.*—Practically all persons are susceptible; permanent acquired immunity is usual after attack. Babies born of mothers who have had the disease are ordinarily immune for the first few months of life.

8. *Occurrence.*—Common in childhood; probably 80 to 90% of persons surviving to age 20 years have had measles; few persons go through life without an attack. Endemic and relatively mild in large metropolitan communities, attaining epidemic proportions about every other year. In smaller communities, and in rural areas outbreaks tend to be wider spaced and somewhat more severe. In areas previously free, or in isolated settlements with long intervals between outbreaks, measles often affects large proportions of the population and fatality is much increased. Prevalent in all seasons except summer, but primarily spring.

9. *Methods of control:*

A. Preventive measures:

1. Education as to special danger of exposing young children to those exhibiting any fever or acute catarrhal symptoms, particularly during years and seasons of epidemic measles.

2. Encouragement by health departments and by private physicians of administration of immune serum globulin (gamma globulin) to infants and children under 3 years of age in families where measles occurs. This product carries no hazard of serum hepatitis.

B. Control of the infected individual, contacts, and environment:

1. Report to local health authority: Case report is compulsory in some jurisdictions, optional in others. Early reporting may secure better isolation and adequate care for the underprivileged child and provide opportunity for passive protection of contacts, Class 2B (p. 7).

2. Isolation: Commonly 7 days from rash to protect the patient against added infection and to limit transfer of measles to susceptible contacts, especially those under 3 years of age.

3. Concurrent disinfection: All articles soiled with secretions of nose and throat.

4. Terminal disinfection: Thorough cleaning.

5. Quarantine: Impractical and of no value in large communities. Exclusion of exposed susceptible school children and teachers from school and from all public gatherings until 14 days from last exposure may be justifiable in sparsely settled rural areas. If date of single exposure is reasonably certain, an exposed susceptible child may be allowed to attend school for the first 7 days of incubation. Quarantine of institutions, wards or dormitories

for young children exposed to measles is of value; strict segregation of infants if measles occurs in an institution.

6. Immunization: Administration of gamma globulin, or serum of convalescent patients or of healthy adults who have had measles, to an exposed person within 3 days after first exposure to a known case of measles, will avert the attack in most instances, and almost certainly modify it. Such passive immunity has a maximum duration of 3 weeks. Given between 4 and 6 days after first exposure, there is reasonable chance of modifying severity of attack and the patient probably will acquire the usual lasting immunity to measles; given after the sixth day, little effect is expected. For protection, the dosage of gamma globulin, given shortly after exposure, is 0.1 cc. per pound of body weight, of convalescent or normal human serum, 20–30 cc. intramuscularly; for modification, gamma globulin in amounts of 0.02 cc. per pound of body weight.

7. Investigation of contacts and source of infection: Search for exposed susceptible children under 3 years of age is profitable. Carriers are not known to occur.

8. Specific treatment: None. Complications should be treated with an appropriate antibiotic or with sulfadiazine.

C. Epidemic measures:

1. Daily examination of exposed children and known susceptible adult contacts, with record of body temperature. Susceptible persons exhibiting a rise of temperature of 0.5° C. (0.9° F.) or more should be isolated promptly pending diagnosis.

2. Schools should not be closed nor classes discontinued; daily observation of children by physician or nurse should be provided and sick children promptly removed.

3. Administration of gamma globulin to all susceptibles has value in institutional outbreaks, in checking spread of infection and in reducing fatality; accept no new admissions and exclude visitors under 16 years of age, whether the measles outbreak is in the institution or in the community. Removal of patients during the pre-eruptive period may prevent an outbreak.

D. International measures: None.

MENINGITIS, MENINGOCOCCAL

1. *Identification.*—An acute bacterial infection characterized by sudden onset with fever, intense headache, nausea and often vomiting, signs of meningeal irritation, and frequently a petechial rash. With modern chemotherapy a fatality of 5 to 10% is usual, supplanting the former 40 to 50%; much variation under both endemic and epidemic conditions. Delirium and coma may appear early; occasional fulminating cases (Waterhouse-Friderichsen syndrome) exhibit signs of collapse and shock from onset. Meningococcemia without extension to the meninges is not uncommon and should be suspected in

cases of otherwise unexplained acute febrile illness, particularly if associated with skin eruption and high leucocytosis. Synonym: Cerebrospinal Fever.

Meningococci can usually be cultivated from the blood, the spinal fluid and the nasopharynx. Smears from petechiae may reveal the infectious agent.

Meningococcal meningitis is to be differentiated from meningism, serous meningitis (lymphocytic choriomeningitis, mumps meningo-encephalitis, tuberculous and syphilitic meningitis) and particularly from secondary meningitis due to H. influenzae, pneumococci, staphylococci, hemolytic streptococci and a number of other less common infectious agents.

2. *Etiologic agent.*—Neisseria meningitidis (N. intracellularis), meningo-coccus.

3. *Source and reservoir of infection.*—Discharges from nose and throat of patients or carriers. Carrier prevalence of 25% or more may exist without occurrence of cases. During epidemic periods more than half of a military organization may be healthy carriers of the strain of meningococcus responsible for the epidemic.

4. *Mode of transmission.*—By contact with infected persons, direct and by droplet spread. Indirect transmission through contact with arti-cles freshly soiled with discharges from the respiratory tract of infected persons has little significance because the meningococcus is especially susceptible to chilling and drying.

5. *Incubation period.*—Varies from 2 to 10 days.

6. *Period of communicability.*—Until meningococci are no longer present in discharges from nose and mouth of patients. Meningococci usu-ally disappear from the nasopharynx within 24 hours after admin-istration of appropriate chemotherapeutic or antibiotic agent.

7. *Susceptibility and resistance.*—Susceptibility to the clinical disease is slight as evidenced by the low ratio of cases to carriers. Younger age groups are more susceptible, but the disease may occur at all ages. Type, degree and duration of immunity after attack are unknown; there are no generally accepted methods for inducing immunity artificially.

8. *Occurrence.*—Endemic and epidemic; no limits in geographic distribu-tion; commonly observed in temperate climates, but large epidemics have occurred in hot, dry regions. Sporadic cases occur through-out the year in both urban and rural areas, with greatest incidence during winter and spring. The disease exhibits high incidence at irregular intervals, with epidemic waves usually lasting 2 to 3 years. In adults, more common where living conditions are crowded; in barracks and institutions.

9. *Methods of control:*

   A. Preventive measures:

      1. Education as to personal cleanliness and necessity of avoid-ing direct contact and droplet infection.

      2. Prevention of overcrowding in living quarters, public trans-portation, working places and especially in barracks, camps and ships.

   B. Control of the infected individual, contacts and environment:

      1. Report to local health authority: Obligatory case report in most states and countries, Class 2A (p. 7).

2. Isolation: Until recovery from acute illness.
3. Concurrent disinfection: Of discharges from the nose and throat and of articles soiled therewith.
4. Terminal disinfection: Cleaning.
5. Quarantine: No complete quarantine; surveillance is profitable.
6. Immunization: None.
7. Investigation of contacts and source of infection: Impracticable.
8. Specific treatment: Sulfadiazine by mouth in an initial loading dose and smaller amounts thereafter; if vomiting is severe, solution of sodium sulfadiazine intravenously after proper hydration. Penicillin in large doses or the tetracyclines may be used in addition.

C. Epidemic measures:
1. Increase the separation of individuals and the ventilation of living and sleeping quarters for such groups of people as are especially exposed to infection because of occupation or some necessity of living condition.
2. If a community—civil, industrial, or military—is suffering unusual risk of infection and the general administration of chemoprophylaxis to exposed persons under medical supervision is practicable, sulfadiazine will lower markedly the carrier rate and limit the spread of the disease (0.5 gm. twice daily for children, 1 gm. twice daily for adults, in both instances for 2 days.

D. International measures: None.

MONILIASIS

1. *Identification.*—The clinical reaction to this fungus infection varies according to location of lesions, allergic state of the patient, and other factors. Common manifestations are thrush, vaginitis or vulvovaginitis, skin lesions of various kinds, bronchopulmonary disease, meningitis and rare generalized infection. Skin and local infections are benign; systemic infections highly fatal. Synonyms: Candidiasis, Thrush.

Identification is difficult and depends upon repeated microscopic demonstration of budding and mycelial forms in direct smears of lesions; fungi may be found in sputum from patients with tuberculosis, other lung infections or tumors. The fungus can be cultured.

2. *Etiologic agent.*—Candida albicans (Monilia albicans).

3. *Source and reservoir of infection.*—Skin and gastrointestinal tract of apparently normal persons. Commonly found in fowls and other animals.

4. *Mode of transmission.*—Probably from auto-inoculation; rarely transmitted from man to man.

5. *Incubation period.*—Unknown.

6. *Period of communicability.*—Unknown.

7. *Susceptibility and resistance.*—Inapparent infections are common. Most adults are hypersensitive to the fungus and possess antibodies. Second attacks are common; clinical manifestations are likely to follow general or local lowering of resistance. Infections of fingers is associated with maceration through long exposure to water (bartenders, housewives). Skin lesions are common in obese people with excessive perspiration in frictional folds, in diabetics and in lactating women. Thrush occurs in debilitated infants, and in older people with ill-fitting dentures. The fungus is frequently found in patients receiving wide spectrum antibiotic therapy.

8. *Occurrence.*—World-wide and sporadic. Clinical infection of adults is more frequent than of children, excluding infants. More common in females than in males.

9. *Methods of control:*

    A. Preventive measures: None.

    B. Control of the infected individual, contacts and environment:

        1. Report to local health authority: Official report ordinarily not justifiable, Class 5 (p. 7).
        2. Isolation: None.
        3. Concurrent disinfection: None.
        4. Terminal disinfection: None.
        5. Quarantine: None.
        6. Immunization: None.
        7. Investigation of contacts and source of infection: Not profitable.
        8. Specific treatment: None. Infections developing during antibiotic therapy sometimes disappear when medication is discontinued.

    C. Epidemic measures: Not applicable.

    D. International measures: None.

MONONUCLEOSIS, INFECTIOUS

1. *Identification.*—An acute infection with irregular clinical manifestations usually accompanied by characteristic lymphocytosis and heterophile antibodies in the blood. Three common clinical entities have been described having one or both characteristics: (1) Glandular fever (Pfeiffer)—enlargement of lymphatic glands and spleen without throat manifestations; common in children; (2) Infectious mononucleosis—continued fever with absent or inconsequential glandular swelling or throat symptoms; common in young adults; (3) Monocytic angina—a characteristic involvement of throat structures with or without lymphatic gland involvement; common in older children and young adults. A rash of variable morphology is an irregular occurrence and jaundice and meningoencephalitis are sometimes seen. The disease rarely ends fatally.

    Laboratory aids to diagnosis are through examination of blood smears and test for heterophile antibodies. Serologic tests for syphilis may be temporarily positive.

2. *Etiologic agent.*—Unknown.

3. *Source of infection.*—Unknown.

4. *Mode of transmission.*—Unknown; the suggestion is of person-to-person transmission.

5. *Incubation period.*—Unknown; seemingly varies from 4 to 14 or more days.

6. *Period of communicability.*—Undetermined.

7. *Susceptibility and resistance.*—Susceptibility apparently general, but incidence greatest among children and young adults. Mild unrecognized cases probably occur. The degree of immunity conferred by an attack is undetermined.

8. *Occurrence.*—Reported from many parts of the world, particularly Continental Europe, Great Britain, Australia and the United States. Observed as isolated cases and in epidemics and probably much more prevalent and more widely distributed than indicated by reported cases. Epidemics are most frequently recognized in schools and institutions for children; cases are commonly reported among medical students, nurses and hospital personnel.

9. *Methods of control:*

   A. Preventive measures: None.

   B. Control of the infected individual, contacts and environment:
      1. Report to local health authority: Obligatory report of epidemics; no individual case report, Class 4 (p. 7).
      2. Isolation: None.
      3. Concurrent disinfection: Of articles soiled with nose and throat discharges.
      4. Terminal disinfection: None.
      5. Quarantine: None.
      6. Immunization: None.
      7. Investigation of contacts and source of infection: For the individual case, of little value.
      8. Specific treatment: None.

   C. Epidemic measures: Field investigation of epidemics should be undertaken with the hope of adding to knowledge of the disease.

   D. International measures: None.

MUMPS

1. *Identification.*—An acute viral infection of sudden onset characterized by fever and by swelling and tenderness of one or more of the salivary glands, usually of the parotid, sometimes of the sublingual or submaxillary glands. Involvement of ovaries and testicles is more frequent in persons past puberty; involvement of the central nervous system is not infrequent early or late in the course of the disease. Orchitis and meningoencephalitis due to mumps virus may occur without involvement of a salivary gland. Death from mumps is exceedingly rare. Synonym: Infectious Parotitis.

   Hemagglutination and complement fixation tests are of value in recognizing atypical forms of infection. The virus may be found in the saliva, blood and cerebrospinal fluid.

2. *Etiologic agent.*—The virus of mumps.

3. *Source and reservoir of infection.*—Saliva of infected persons.

4. *Mode of transmission.*—By droplet spread and by direct contact with an infected person or with articles freshly soiled with the saliva of such persons.

5. *Incubation period.*—From 12 to 26 days, commonly 18 days.

6. *Period of communicability.*—From about 2 days before distinctive symptoms and persisting as much as 9 days thereafter, but no longer than swelling of a salivary gland. Susceptibles may contract the disease through exposure to persons with inapparent infection.

7. *Susceptibility and resistance.*—Susceptibility believed to be general. Second attacks are uncommon; immunity generally held to be life-long; develops after inapparent as well as clinical attack. An allergic tuberculin-like response occurs when inactivated virus is injected intradermally in persons previously infected.

8. *Occurrence.*—Clinical disease is less frequent than with other common communicable diseases of childhood such as measles and chickenpox; many inapparent infections. Winter and spring are seasons of greatest prevalence; sporadic and epidemic except in large cities, where it is endemic. Outbreaks occur more frequently and are more serious in aggregations of young people, especially military.

9. *Methods of control:*

   A. Preventive measures: None.

   B. Control of the infected individual, contacts and environment:

   1. Report to local health authority: Official report not ordinarily justifiable, Class 5 (p. 7).
   2. Isolation: Until swelling of salivary glands has subsided.
   3. Concurrent disinfection: Of eating and drinking utensils; of articles soiled with secretions of nose and throat.
   4. Terminal disinfection: None.
   5. Quarantine: None.
   6. Immunization: None.
   7. Investigation of contacts and source of infection: Not profitable.
   8. Specific treatment: None.

   C. Epidemic measures: No procedures in common use can be relied upon as a means of effective control of the disease or of epidemics. Active immunization by vaccines is experimental.

   D. International measures: None.

NOCARDIOSIS

1. *Identification.*—A chronic fungus infection, frequently initiated in the lungs, with hematogenous spread to produce peritonitis, meningitis, brain abscess and other pyogenic processes; highly fatal. A localized fungus tumor or mycetoma, usually of a lower extremity, is a common, more benign but highly disabling form of the disease.

   Microscopic examination of stained smears of sputum, pus or spinal fluid and of "granules" of mycetomas aids in diagnosis; confirmation by culture and pathogenicity for animals.

   Mycetomas caused by a variety of fungi other than Nocardia often are referred to as maduramycosis (Madura foot); they require differentiation.

2. *Etiologic agent.*—Nocardia asteroides. Other species of Nocardia also cause mycetomas.

3. *Source and reservoir of infection.*—Unknown; presumably soil.

4. *Mode of transmission.*—Direct contact with contaminated soil through minor traumatic wounds and abrasions; pulmonary infections presumably through inhalation of organisms suspended in dust-contaminated air. Not directly transmissible in nature from man to man.

5. *Incubation period.*—Unknown; probably weeks or months.

6. *Period of communicability.*—Unknown.

7. *Susceptibility and resistance.*—Susceptibility is probably general; no immunity after attack.

8. *Occurrence.*—Occasional sporadic infections in all parts of the world. Mycetomas are more common in regions where people go barefoot. No evidence of age, sex or racial differences.

9. *Methods of control:*

    A. Preventive measures: None.

    B. Control of the infected individual, contacts and environment:

        1. Report to local health authority: Official report not ordinarily justifiable, Class 5 (p. 7).

        2. Isolation: None.

        3. Concurrent disinfection: Of discharges and contaminated dressings.

        4. Terminal disinfection: Thorough cleaning.

        5. Quarantine: None.

        6. Immunization: None.

        7. Investigation of contacts and source of infection: Not profitable.

        8. Specific treatment: Sulfonamides and penicillin are effective in systemic infections if given early and for prolonged periods.

    C. Epidemic measures: Not applicable, a sporadic disease.

    D. International measures: None.

ONCHOCERCIASIS

1. *Identification.*—A chronic non-fatal disease caused by a filarial worm which forms fibrous nodules in skin and subcutaneous tissues, particularly of head and shoulders (America) or around the waist (Africa). The female discharges microfilariae which migrate through the skin, and if on the head, often reach the eye, leading to ocular disturbances and sometimes blindness. Skin surrounding nodules may become indurated, pigmented and inflamed.

    Laboratory diagnosis is by superficial biopsy of skin with demonstration of microfilariae in fresh tissue by microscopic examination; by excision of nodule and finding adult worms; in ocular manifestations, by observation with ophthalmic microscope of microfilariae in the eye.

2. *Etiologic agent.*—Onchocerca volvulus, a filarial nematode worm.

3. *Source and reservoir of infection.*—Immediate source is the blackfly; reservoir is infected persons with microfilariae in the skin.

4. *Mode of transmission.*—By the bite of infected blackflies of the genus Simulium; in Guatemala and Mexico S. ochraceum, S. callidum, S. metallicum and possibly other species; in Africa S. damnosum and probably S. neavei. The microfilariae penetrate the thoracic muscles of the vector, develop into infective larvae, migrate to the proboscis and are liberated on the skin of man as the insect feeds; vector is infectious after 6 days or longer.

5. *Incubation period.*—Nodules may be visible 3 to 4 months after infection. Worms begin to discharge larvae 1 year or more after infection.

6. *Period of Communicability.*—As long as living microfilariae persist in the skin; many months, probably years.

7. *Susceptibility and resistance.*—Susceptibility is general.

8. *Occurrence.*—Geographical distribution in western hemisphere limited to Guatemala (principally Western slope of continental divide), southern Mexico (states of Chiapas and Oaxaca), and northeast Venezuela; in Africa along west coast from Sierra Leone south to the Belgian Congo, and eastward through the Congo to the French and British Sudan, Uganda, Nyasaland, and Kenya. In some localities, one half or more of the population is infected.

9. *Methods of control:*

    A. Preventive measures:

        1. Avoid bites of Simulium flies by covering body and head as much as possible, or by use of insect repellents.

        2. Control of vector larvae in rapidly running streams and in artificial waterways by DDT or other insecticide with residual effect.

        3. Provision of facilities for diagnosis and treatment.

    B. Control of the infected individual, contacts and environment:

        1. Report to local health authority: In selected endemic areas; in most countries not a reportable disease, Class 3C (p. 7).

        2. Isolation: None.

        3. Concurrent disinfection: None.

        4. Terminal disinfection: None.

        5. Quarantine: None.

        6. Immunization: None.

        7. Investigation of contacts and source of infection: A community problem (see 9A, 9C).

        8. Specific treatment: Treatment with surinan sodium (naphuride sodium, Bayer 205) leads to gradual disappearance of microfilariae and kills worms. Undesirable reactions may occur. Diethylcarbamazine (hetrazan) is not recommended because of severe reactions due to destruction of larvae, and absence of lethal action on adult worms. Excision of developing nodules in order to eliminate adult worms.

    C. Epidemic measures: In areas of high prevalence make concerted effort to reduce incidence, using measures listed under 9A.

    D. International measures: Coordinated programs entered into by neighboring countries where the disease is endemic, designed to prevent migration of infected persons across international boundaries and to institute treatment and other control measures near such boundaries.

PARAGONIMIASIS

1. *Identification.*—A trematode infection, with clinical manifestations in man dependent upon path of migration and organs parasitized. The lungs are the more frequent site, where worms are surrounded by an inflammatory reaction which eventually organizes into a fibrous cystic lesion. Clinical symptoms are cough and hemoptysis; in many cases roentgenographic findings closely simulate pulmonary tuberculosis. Ectopic development is not infrequent, worms maturing in such sites as the intestine, lymph glands, genito-urinary tract, subcutaneous tissue and brain, the latter often associated with a Jacksonian-type epilepsy. Infections are usually chronic, lasting for many years, and patients may appear surprisingly well. Synonyms: Pulmonary Distomiasis, Endemic Hemoptysis, Oriental Liver Fluke Disease.

   The sputum generally contains flecks of orange-brown pigment sometimes diffusely distributed, in which masses of worm eggs are seen microscopically. Eggs are also found in feces; rarely in urine.

2. *Etiologic agent.*—Paragonimus westermani.

3. *Source and reservoir of infection.*—Crabs and crayfish, second intermediate hosts, are the immediate source of infection. Humans and other mammals harboring the adult fluke are reservoirs.

4. *Mode of transmission.*—Eggs leave the definitive host via sputum and feces, gain entrance to fresh water, and embryonate in 2 to 4 weeks. A larva (miracidium) hatches, and on penetrating a suitable fresh water snail (Semisulcospira, Orient; Pomatiopsis, North America) undergoes a cycle of development which requires approximately 3 months. Larvae (cercariae) emerge from the snail, and penetrate and encyst in fresh water crabs (Eriocheir and Potamon, Orient) and crayfish (Astacus, Orient; Cambarus, North America). When the flesh of crustacea containing infective larvae (metacercariae) is ingested by a susceptible mammal raw or only partially cooked, the larva emerges in the duodenum, penetrates into the abdominal cavity, migrates through the diaphragm into the thoracic cavity, penetrates the pleura and develops in lung parenchyma into an egg-producing adult. Worms occasionally develop to maturity in various other organs. In addition to man, the dog, cat, pig, and wild carnivores may act as definitive hosts.

5. *Incubation period.*—Flukes mature and begin to lay eggs approximately 6 weeks after man ingests infective larvae. The interval until symptoms appear is long, variable and poorly defined.

6. *Period of communicability.*—Eggs may be discharged by the human host for as long as 20 years or more. Little available information on duration of infection in mollusk and crustacean hosts.

7. *Susceptibility and resistance.*—Susceptibility is general. Increased resistance possibly develops as a result of infection.

8. *Occurrence.*—Extensive in the Far East, particularly Korea, Japan, Formosa, the Philippines, and parts of China. Scattered foci in Africa, India, and parts of South America. P. kellicotti, a closely related form found in North America, supposedly has infected man once.

9. *Methods of control:*

    A. Preventive measures:

        1. Education of people in endemic areas concerning the life cycle of the parasite; stress thorough cooking of crustacea.

        2. Prohibition by law of sale of crabs has had some result in Korea.

        3. Sanitary disposal of sputum and feces.

        4. Control of snails with proper molluscacides is feasible in some areas, as well as destruction of crabs.

    B. Control of the infected individual, contacts and environment:

        1. Report to local health authority: In selected endemic areas; in most countries not a reportable disease, Class 3B (p. 7).

        2. Isolation: None.

        3. Concurrent disinfection: Of sputum and feces.

        4. Terminal disinfection: None.

        5. Quarantine: None.

        6. Immunization: None.

        7. Investigation of contacts and source of infection: Within the immediate premises, usually unproductive; a community problem (see 9C).

        8. Specific treatment: None; emetine hydrochloride causes temporary amelioration of symptoms and cessation of egg excretion but is not curative.

    C. Epidemic measures: In an endemic area, occurrence of small clusters of cases or even sporadic infections is important indication for examination of local waters for infected snails, crabs and crayfish, and determination of reservoir mammalian hosts.

    D. International measures: None.

PARATYPHOID FEVER

1. *Identification.*—A generalized bacterial infection with continued fever and involvement of lymphoid tissues of intestines, enlargement of spleen, sometimes rose spots on trunk, usually diarrhea. Many mild infections give no more than a transient diarrhea. Fatality is much less than for typhoid fever.

    Paratyphoid bacilli may be found in feces, blood, and urine.

2. *Etiologic agent.*—Salmonella paratyphi, S. schottmuelleri, S. hirschfeldi; Paratyphoid bacilli, A, B, and C.

3. *Source and reservoir of infection.*—Feces and urine of patients or carriers, with temporary carriers often frequent in epidemics.

4. *Mode of transmission.*—Direct or indirect contact with patient or carrier. Vehicles of indirect spread are food, especially milk, milk products and shellfish, usually contaminated by hands of a carrier or missed case. Under some conditions, flies are vectors. Few outbreaks are related to water supplies. Most large outbreaks in England in recent years have been associated with synthetic cream.

5. *Incubation period.*—One to 10 days; somewhat longer for paratyphoid A than for B and C.

6. *Period of communicability.*—As long as paratyphoid bacilli appear in excreta; usually from appearance of prodromal symptoms, throughout illness and for varying periods after recovery.

7. *Susceptibility and resistance.*—Susceptibility is general. A high degree of resistance usually follows recovery. The degree of protection conferred by paratyphoid vaccine is uncertain.

8. *Occurrence.*—Incidence in United States has fallen with that of typhoid fever. Occurs sporadically or in limited outbreaks due to contact or to contaminated food, milk or water. Probably more common than reports suggest due to large number of unrecognized infections. Paratyphoid A infection is rare in United States, but common in Europe; paratyphoid B is common in the United States, often as a transient diarrhea of undetermined etiology; both are still frequent in countries where sanitation is defective. Paratyphoid C infection is extremely rare in United States but common in Eastern Europe and Asia.

9. *Methods of control:*

    A. Preventive measures:

        1. The preventive measures applicable to paratyphoid fever are those listed under Typhoid Fever 9A, p. 202.

    B. Control of the infected individual, contacts and environment:

        1. Report to local health authority: Obligatory case report in most states and countries, both suspect and confirmed infections, Class 2A (p. 7).

        2. Items 2–8 of Typhoid Fever, 9B, pp. 202, 203 also apply to paratyphoid fever. Therapeutic results from chloramphenicol are not striking.

    C. Epidemic measures:

        1. The procedures are those of Typhoid Fever 9C, p. 203.

    D. International measures: Inoculation of international travellers with triple typhoid vaccine (TAB, typhoid, paratyphoid A, paratyphoid B) is advisable for travel in all areas except the United States, Canada, Great Britain and Northwest Europe, if not protected through previous attack.

PEDICULOSIS

1. *Identification.*—Infestation with adult lice, larvae or nits, of the scalp, of the hairy parts of the body, or of clothing, especially along the seams of inner surfaces. Synonym: Lousiness.

2. *Infesting agents.*—Pediculus humanus, head louse or body louse, and Phthirus pubis, crab louse.

3. *Source of infestation.*—Infested persons or their personal belongings, particularly body clothing; infested beds.

4. *Mode of transmission.*—Direct contact with an infested person and indirectly by contact with clothing and headgear of such persons.

4. *Incubation period.*—Under optimum conditions, the eggs hatch in a week, and sexual maturity is reached in approximately 2 weeks.

6. *Period of communicability.*—While lice remain alive on the infested person or in his clothing, and until eggs (nits) in hair and clothing have been destroyed.

7. *Susceptibility and resistance.*—Any person may become lousy under suitable conditions of exposure. Repeated infestations often result in dermal hypersensitivity.

8. *Occurrence.*—Cosmopolitan. The head louse is common in outbreaks among school children.

9. *Methods of control:*

   A. Preventive measures:

      1. Direct inspection of the heads and, when necessary, of the body and clothing where lousiness is found in groups of children or adults, particularly of children in schools, institutions and camp groups.

      2. Education in the value of using hot water and soap to maintain cleanliness, and laundering of clothing to destroy nits and lice.

      3. Provision of residual insecticide for freeing persons and clothing of lice. (See 9B8.)

   B. Control of the infested individual, contacts and environment:

      1. Report to local health authority: Official report not ordinarily justifiable; school authorities should be informed, Class 5 (p. 7).

      2. Isolation: Not necessary after application of effective insecticide.

      3. Concurrent disinfestation: Of other members of family or associated group.

      4. Terminal disinfestation: None.

      5. Quarantine: None.

      6. Immunization: Does not apply.

      7. Investigation of contacts and source of infestation: Examination of household and other close personal contacts.

      8. Specific treatment: 10% DDT dusting powder for body and head lice; dust clothing, particularly along seams, and the hair; cover head with towel or cap for several hours; comb hair with fine tooth comb; repeat dusting in one week without washing hair or clothing in the interim. For crab lice, dust hairy parts of body and bathe after 12 to 24 hours; repeat treatment in one week; continue treatment at weekly intervals until lice or nits are no longer present. In parts of Korea and Egypt lice are known to have become DDT-resistant; gamma isomer of benzene hexachloride (lindane) may then be substituted as a dusting powder.

   C. Epidemic measures: Mass treatment as recommended in 9B8.

   D. International measures: None.

PEMPHIGUS NEONATORUM

1. *Identification.*—An acute vesicular or bullous eruption of the skin of newborn infants, particularly in nurseries. Onset is commonly between the 4th and 10th day of life as vesicles or bullae, usually first seen on the lower abdomen but spreading to the skin of any part of the body. Vesicles rupture, thin crusts form, and new lesions develop, tending to spread peripherally and often coalescing. Constitutional symptoms are unusual but if lesions are widespread, fever, diarrhea and a complicating pneumonia, meningitis or bacteremia may occur. Death sometimes follows. Synonym: Impetigo of the Newborn.

2. *Etiologic agent.*—Probably staphylococci, in frequent association with streptococci.

3. *Source and reservoir of infection.*—Infected infants, attendants or visitors.

4. *Mode of transmission.*—By direct contact with the skin of infected infants or with articles freshly contaminated with discharges from lesions; also by contact with other individuals whose skin is infected or contaminated with the infectious agents.

5. *Incubation period.*—Two to 5 days.

6. *Period of communicability.*—Until the lesions have healed; usually about 1 or 2 weeks.

7. *Susceptibility and resistance.*—Susceptibility of newborn infants is general. Immunity does not follow an attack.

8. *Occurrence.*—Chiefly in nurseries for the newborn, particularly in association with laxness in nursing technics and much handling of infants. Incidence highest in countries such as the United States, where percentage of deliveries in hospitals is high and newborn infants are housed in nurseries. Occurs in all seasons of the year.

9. *Methods of control:*

   A. Preventive measures: Cleanliness is the most important preventive measure. The infant should be handled as little as possible. Excess vernix should be wiped gently from the scalp and face, and no water or oil bath given until ready for discharge. Examination by physicians should be at a minimum. Infants should be weighed not more than twice a week and temperature taken not oftener than once a day. Nurses and attendants should wash their hands with soap and water after diapering and before feeding an infant; those with infections of the skin should be excluded from care of infants. Visitors should not be permitted in nurseries. Scrupulous attention must be given to aseptic precautions, and to bedding, furnishings, gowns and masks of attendants.

   B. Control of the infected individual, contacts and environment:

      1. Report to local health authority: Obligatory report of epidemics; no individual case report, Class 4 (p. 7). Any case in a hospital or other nursery is to be interpreted as a potential epidemic. Willful attempt to delay control measures by labelling cases as dermatitis or folliculitis is a common source of trouble.

      2. Isolation: Prompt isolation of infected infants.

3. Concurrent disinfection: Collect and burn dressings; launder separately bedding and clothing of patients.
4. Terminal disinfection: Wash nursery, cribs and other furniture with soap and water after all infants have been discharged; boil instruments and basins, and sterilize mattresses.
5. Quarantine: Of all exposed newborn infants.
6. Immunization: None.
7. Investigation of contacts and source of infection: Examine nurses and attendants for presence of skin lesions.
8. Specific treatment: Ammoniated mercury ointment or gentian violet solution or penicillin ointment. If lesions are widespread, use penicillin intramuscularly. ACTH or cortisone gives temporary relief in severe cases.

C. Epidemic measures:
   1. If an outbreak (more than 1 case) occurs in a nursery, isolate all patients and quarantine contacts until all have been discharged. Permit no new admissions to quarantined nursery.
   2. Exclude nurses and attendants with skin infections.
   3. Investigate adequacy of nursing procedures; emphasize cleanliness and personal hygiene.
   4. Nursing staffs of isolation and quarantined nurseries should not work in nurseries housing normal newborn infants.

D. International measures: None.

PERTUSSIS

1. *Identification.*—An acute bacterial infection involving trachea, bronchi and bronchioles, and characterized by a typical cough, usually of one to two months duration. The initial catarrhal stage has an insidious onset with irritating cough, which gradually becomes paroxysmal, usually within one to two weeks. Paroxysms are characterized by a repeated series of violent coughs, each series having many coughs without intervening inhalation and followed by characteristic crowing or high pitched inspiratory whoop; frequently ends with expulsion of clear, tenacious mucus. Young infants and adults often do not have the typical paroxysm. An absolute lymphocytosis is usually present. The overall case fatality is low, less than 0.5%, but approximately 85% of deaths and 15% of cases are among children aged less than 2 years. Synonym: Whooping Cough.

The etiologic agent is readily recovered during catarrhal and early paroxysmal stages by nasopharyngeal swab. Bacteriological characteristics differentiate infections with Haemophilus parapertussis which is immunologically distinct from H. pertussis.

2. *Etiologic agent.*—Hemophilus pertussis. Pertussis bacillus.

3. *Source and reservoir of infection.*—Discharges from the laryngeal and bronchial mucous membranes of infected persons.

4. *Mode of transmission.*—By direct contact with an infected person, by droplet spread or indirectly by contact with articles freshly soiled with discharges of such persons.

5. *Incubation period.*—Commonly 7 days, almost uniformly within 10 days, and not exceeding 21 days.

6. *Period of communicability.*—Particularly communicable in early catarrhal stage before paroxysmal cough confirms provisional clinical
   diagnosis. After paroxysms are established communicability gradually decreases and becomes negligible for ordinary non-familial
   contacts in about 3 weeks even though spasmodic cough with
   whoop may persist. For control purposes, the communicable stage
   is considered to extend from 7 days after exposure to 3 weeks after
   onset of typical paroxysms.

7. *Susceptibility and resistance.*—Susceptibility is general; no good evidence of temporary passive immunity in young infants born of immune mothers. Pertussis is predominantly a childhood disease, the
   incidence being highest under seven years of age and mortality
   highest in infants, particularly those under six months. One attack confers a definite and prolonged immunity but second attacks
   occasionally occur, particularly in exposed adults. Fatality is
   higher in females than males at all ages. Both active and passive
   artificial immunity may be induced by appropriate means.

8. Occurrence.—A frequent and common disease among children every
   where regardless of race, climate, or geographic location. In large
   communities the incidence is generally higher in late winter and
   early spring; in smaller communities the seasonal incidence is
   variable.

9. *Methods of control:*

   A. Preventive measures:

      1. General immunization of all susceptible pre-school children
         is an effective procedure for control of pertussis. Plain
         or alum adjuvant vaccines may be used either alone or
         in combination with diphtheria and tetanus toxoids.
         Three doses of an alum adjuvant vaccine mixed with
         diphtheria and generally tetanus toxoid, administered at
         four-week intervals, beginning at 2 to 6 months of age,
         is commonly used in the United States for simultaneous
         immunization against all three diseases. In general,
         routine immunization can be started at 3 to 4 months
         of age. The need for subsequent reinforcing doses of
         pertussis vaccine is not definitely established but when
         primary immunization is properly carried out in infancy,
         a single reinforcing dose is generally advised at 1 to 2
         and again at 4 to 5 years of age; in addition, under cir-
         cumstances of known direct exposure through familial
         contact. Infants living in institutions and in households
         with other susceptible children, particularly during the
         months when pertussis is prevalent in the community,
         should have active immunization started by the time they
         are 2 months of age.

      2. Educational measures to inform the public and particularly
         parents of infants of the dangers of pertussis and of the
         advantages of immunization in infancy.

   B. Control of the infected individual, contacts and environment:

      1. Report to local health authority: Case report obligatory in
         most states and countries, Class 2B (p. 7).

      2. Isolation: Separation of the patient from susceptible children
         and exclusion of the patient from school and public places
         for the recognized period of communicability. Isolation

of children over 2 years of age is often impracticable; even for those under 2, should not be insisted upon at the expense of fresh air in the open if weather permits.

3. Concurrent disinfection: Discharges from the nose and throat and articles soiled therewith.

4. Terminal disinfection: Thorough cleaning.

5. Quarantine: Limited to exclusion of non-immune children from school and public gatherings for 14 days after last exposure to a household or similar case; may be omitted if exposed non-immune children are seen by a physician or nurse on arrival at school each day for 14 days after last exposure. Particularly important to protect children under 3 years against contact with known or suspected whooping cough.

6. Immunization: Brief and relative passive immunity may be conveyed to young children by administration of appropriate amounts of hyperimmune or convalescent serum. The risk of homologous serum jaundice from use of human serum must be kept in mind. Artificial active immunization after effective exposure is of no proven value.

7. Investigation of contacts and source of infection: Carriers in the exact sense of the term are not known; search for missed and atypical cases among contacts.

8. Specific treatment: None; convalescent serum, serum from immunized donors, and similar agents appear to help when given early in severe cases. The tetracycline antibiotics and probably chloramphenicol tend to abort the infection, but not the symptoms, although minor amelioration may follow.

C. Epidemic measures: A search for unrecognized and unreported cases is of value to protect young children from exposure and to assure adequate medical care for those exposed, especially infants. The comparatively high mortality in young infants justifies intensive effort toward their protection.

D. International measures:

1. Active immunization of susceptible infants and young children travelling to other countries, if not already protected, with attention to desirable reinforcing dose.

PHLEBOTOMUS FEVER

1. *Identification.*—A 3 or 4 day fever clinically not unlike influenza except for absence of inflammation of the respiratory tract. Headache, fever of 38.3° C. to 38.9° C. (101° F. to 102° F.), retrobulbar pain on motion of the eyes, injected sclerae, malaise, and pain in the limbs and back are characteristic. Leucopenia is usual, most prominent on 4th or 5th day after onset of fever. Temperature is occasionally higher and the disease may present alarming symptoms but death is rare. Diagnosis is clinical and epidemiological through occurrence of multiple and similar cases. Synonyms: Pappataci Fever, Sandfly Fever.

Diagnosis may be confirmed by neutralization test, using mouse adapted virus.

2. *Etiologic agent.*—The virus of phlebotomus fever.

3. *Source and reservoir of infection.*—The immediate source of infection in an infected Phlebotomus. The infected person is one reservoir; the existence of an added animal reservoir, is suspected but not demonstrated.

4. *Mode of transmission.*—The vector is a small, hairy, blood-sucking midge, Phlebotomus papatasii, the common sandfly, which bites at night and has a limited flight range; other species of Phlebotomus may carry the virus.

5. *Incubation period.*—Up to 6 days, usually 3 to 4 days, rarely less.

6. *Period of communicability.*—Virus is present in the blood of an infected person at least 24 hours before and 24 hours after onset of fever. Phlebotomus becomes infective about 7 days after biting an infected person and remains so for life.

7. *Susceptibility and resistance.*—Susceptibility is essentially universal, acquired immunity lasting. Relative resistance of native populations in sandfly areas is probably attributable to infection early in life.

8. *Occurrence.*—In those parts of Europe, Africa, and Asia where the vector exists; not recognized with certainty in Central or South America. A disease of subtropical and tropical areas with long periods of hot, dry weather, in general a belt extending around the Mediterranean and eastward into Burma and China. Seasonal, between April and October, and prone to appear as a disease of troops and travellers from non-endemic areas.

9. *Methods of control:*

   A. Preventive measures:

      1. Control of sandflies is the important consideration. For detailed procedures, see Bartonellosis, p. 27.

   B. Control of the infected individual, contacts and environment:

      1. Report to local health authority: In selected endemic areas; in most countries not a reportable disease, Class 3C (p. 7).

      2. Isolation: None; protect infected individual from bites of Phlebotomus for first few days of illness, by screening or mosquito bed nets (25–30 mesh to the inch) or by spraying quarters with insecticide having residual action; if not possible, killing of Phlebotomus flies in living quarters may be helpful.

      3. Concurrent disinfection: None; destruction of sandflies in the dwelling.

      4. Terminal disinfection: None.

      5. Quarantine: None.

      6. Immunization: None currently available.

      7. Investigation of contacts and source of infection: Search for breeding areas of sandflies around dwellings, especially in rubble heaps, masonry cracks, and under stones.

      8. Specific treatment: None.

C. Epidemic measures:
1. Community use of insecticide to destroy the Phlebotomus midge in and about human habitations.
2. Educational publicity designed to inform the people of the conditions under which infection is acquired and to enlist their cooperation with public authorities in efforts to eliminate the Phlebotomus and to avoid its bite by the use of repellents while in infected areas, particularly after sundown.

D. International measures: None.

PINTA

1. *Identification.*—An acute and chronic non-venereal treponematosis, characterized clinically by a superficial non-ulcerative primary lesion, a secondary eruption, and late dyschromic changes in the skin. Within 7 to 20 days after inoculation a non-ulcerating scaling papule appears, usually on hands, legs or dorsum of feet, and having a satellite bubo. In 5 to 12 months a macular, papular, erythemato-squamous secondary rash appears and may evolve into tertiary lesions, the dyschromic stage, with achromic or pigmented (blue, pink, yellow, violet) spots of variable size, mainly on distal portions of extremities but often including trunk and face. In rare instances the untreated disease may end fatally. Synonyms: Mal del Pinto, Carate, Tina, Lota, Empeines, Azul, and others.

Serologic tests for syphilis usually become reactive during the secondary rash and thereafter behave as in venereal syphilis.

2. *Etiologic agent.*—Treponema carateum.

3. *Source and reservoir of infection.*—Infected persons; principally initial skin lesions and those of early dyschromic stage.

4. *Mode of transmission.*—Unknown; evidence suggests transmission by direct and indirect contact; location of primary lesions suggests an influence by trauma. Various biting and sucking arthropods have been implicated; rare reports of venereal and congenital transmission.

5. *Incubation period.*—7 to 20 days.

6. *Period of communicability.*—Unknown; potentially communicable while skin lesions are active, sometimes for several years.

7. *Susceptibility and resistance.*—Undefined; presumably as in other treponematoses. Rare in white persons, suggesting some inherent insusceptibility, but not distinguished clearly from factors of personal hygiene and social and economic status.

8. *Occurrence.*—Frequent among dark-skinned people of tropics and subtropics; in Western Hemisphere among Negroes, native Indians and those of mixed blood. Pinta-like conditions are reported from east and west coasts of Africa, North Africa, the Middle East, and in India and the Philippines. Predominantly a disease of childhood.

9. *Methods of control:*

A. Preventive measures: Those applicable to other treponematoses apply to pinta. See Yaws 9A (p. 208).

B. Control of the infected individual, contacts and environment:
   1. Report to local health authority: In selected endemic areas; in most countries not a reportable disease, Class 3B (p. 7).
   2. Items 2 to 8, see Yaws 9B (pp. 208, 209).
C. Epidemic measures: See Yaws 9C.
D. International measures: See Yaws 9D.

PLAGUE

1. *Identification.*—A severe and highly fatal disease, characterized by rapid clinical course with high fever, progressive heart failure and nervous symptoms such as loss of coordinating power over voluntary muscles, delirium or coma. Conjunctival injection is common, skin hemorrhages or pustular eruptions may occur. Three clinical forms are recognized: a) The bubonic type is most common; acutely inflamed and painful swellings of lymph nodes draining the site of original inoculation. The infection often progresses to septicemia with localization in any part of the body. Secondary terminal pneumonia is an important complication; b) Primary septicemic plague is rare and probably represents a form of bubonic plague in which the bubo is obscure; c) Primary pneumonic plague is ordinarily uncommon but occurs in localized and sometimes devastating outbreaks among closely associated groups during epidemics of bubonic plague. Bubonic plague has a fatality of 25 to 50% or greater when untreated; primary pneumonic and septicemic forms are usually fatal. Modern methods of therapy reduce these rates, especially for bubonic plague. Synonyms: Pest, Black Death.

   Diagnosis is confirmed by demonstrating the infectious agent in fluid aspirated from buboes, in blood, or in sputum in severe or pneumonic forms.

2. *Etiologic agent.*—Pasteurella pestis, plague bacillus.

3. *Source and reservoir of infection.*—The source of bubonic infection is the flea; in pneumonic plague, exhaled droplets and sputum of patients. The reservoir of plague, and the source of flea infection, is a large series of wild rodents infected in nature in many parts of the world (sylvatic plague or wild rodent plague). The infection is apt to pass over to domestic rodents in large cities, particularly in seaports (urban plague).

4. *Mode of transmission.*—Bubonic plague results from the bite of the infected rat flea, Xenopsylla cheopis and certain other species. Pneumonic plague is spread by person-to-person contact from patients with primary pneumonic plague or from patients with bubonic plague who develop terminal plague pneumonia. Accidental infections may occur among laboratory workers.

5. *Incubation period.*—From 2 to 6 days in bubonic plague; 3 to 4 days in pneumonic plague; may be shorter, rarely longer.

6. *Period of communicability.*—Bubonic plague is not directly communicable from person to person except through terminal plague pneumonia. Fleas remain infective for life, days or weeks, or may clear themselves of the infection. Pneumonic plague may become

intensely communicable under climatic or social conditions which lead to overcrowding in unsanitary dwellings.

7. *Susceptibility and resistance.*—Susceptibility is general. Occasionally bubonic infection remains localized and is of short duration, pestis minor. Immunity after recovery is temporary and relative. Active immunization with a vaccine of killed bacteria may confer considerable protection for some months when administered in 2 or 3 doses at weekly intervals; repeated stimulating injections are necessary for continued protection. Vaccines prepared with living avirulent strains may confer satisfactory immunity in one dose, repeated once yearly.

8. *Occurrence.*—Sylvatic plague exists in the western third of the United States and in large areas in South America, in Central and South Africa, and in the Near East with the center in Iranian Kurdistan. The foci in southeast Russia and in Central Asia are possibly quiescent. The human disease in the United States is confined to rare instances of exposure to wild rodents. Urban plague has been largely controlled throughout most of the world but rural bubonic plague of rat origin continues as a serious health problem in some countries, particularly India, Burma, Indonesia (Java) and China. The threat of re-established urban plague thus continues.

9. *Methods of control:*

   A. Preventive measures:

      1. Periodic surveys in endemic and in potential epidemic areas to determine the prevalence of rats and rat fleas; suppression of rats by poisoning or trapping in urban areas. Continuing inspection and survey of wild rodents and their ectoparasites in areas of sylvatic plague. In areas where plague is present or threatening, systematic search for evidence of infection in rodents and their fleas by pooling methods.

      2. Rat-proofing of buildings and reduction of breeding places and harborages, particularly on docks and in warehouses.

      3. Rat control on ships by rat-proofing or periodic fumigation, combined when necessary with destruction of rats and their fleas in vessels and cargoes arriving from plague localities.

   B. Control of the infected individual, contacts and environment:

      1. Report to local health authority: Case report of suspect and confirmed cases universally required by international regulation, Class 1 (p. 6).

      2. Isolation: Hospitalize all patients if practical; reasonable aseptic precautions for patients with bubonic plague, and strict isolation for primary pneumonic plague or patients developing plague pneumonia.

      3. Concurrent disinfection: Sputum and purulent discharges, and articles soiled therewith; urine and feces of patients.

      4. Terminal disinfection: Thorough cleaning; bodies of persons dying of plague should be handled with strict aseptic precautions.

      5. Quarantine: Contacts of bubonic plague, disinfestation with insecticide powder such as 5–10% DDT in talc or pyrophyllite and surveillance for 6 days; contacts of pneumonic plague, quarantine for 6 days with close surveillance for developing illness; dust with insecticide powder.

6. Immunization: None; the management of contacts is by chemoprophylaxis. For all contacts of pneumonic plague, sulfadiazine, 3 gms daily for 6 days; and similarly for contacts of bubonic plague if risk is judged appreciable. Institute specific therapy immediately if a contact develops fever.

7. Investigation of contacts and source of infection: Search for infected rodents and fleas or exposure to preceding cases of plague pneumonia or pneumonic plague.

   Focal attack on fleas should precede anti-rat measures, using an appropriate insecticide powder with residual effect such as 10 percent DDT in talc or pyrophyllite. Dust rat runs and rat harborages in known or suspected focal areas. Disinfect by dusting or insecticide spray the houses, outhouses and household furnishings in the same areas. Dust the persons and clothing of immediate contacts and all other residents in the immediate vicinity. Supplemental suppression of rat populations by poisoning or trapping then follows.

8. Specific treatment: Streptomycin and the tetracycline antibiotics are highly effective for all forms of plague when used early; results good even in pneumonic plague if therapy is begun within 24 hours of onset, poor later. Recurrence of fever during streptomycin therapy may indicate secondary pneumonia caused by gram positive cocci; in such cases, penicillin should be used with continued streptomycin; penicillin not effective against plague itself. Sulfadiazine should be used if antibiotics are not available; frequently used to continue treatment begun with antibiotics. These drugs are also effective in protection of contacts, sulfadiazine being most used.

C. Epidemic measures:

1. Investigate all deaths, with autopsy and laboratory examinations when indicated. Develop case-finding facilities. Establish the best possible provision for diagnosis and treatment. Alert all existing medical facilities toward immediate reporting and toward utilization of diagnostic and therapy services. Provide adequate laboratory services, and supplies of antibiotics.

2. Institute intensive flea control in expanding circles from known focal areas.

3. Supplemental rat destruction within affected areas.

4. Prophylactic administration of appropriate antibiotics or sulfadiazine to all medical, nursing and public health personnel exposed to risk may be considered; surveillance to detect disease in its earliest stages.

5. Personal protection of field workers against fleas by weekly dusting of clothing with insecticide powder. Daily application of insect repellents is a valuable adjunct.

6. Widespread active immunization of native populations with a single dose of avirulent living plague vaccine has proved valuable. Killed vaccines are less useful in such circumstances because of practical difficulties in administering repeated injections.

D. International measures:
  1. Telegraphic notification of WHO and adjacent countries by governments of the existence of an epidemic of plague.
  2. Measures applicable to ships, aircraft and land transport arriving from plague areas are specified in International Sanitary Regulations (WHO Techn. Rep. Ser. No. 41, Geneva, 1951).
  3. All ships should be periodically deratized, or be permanently kept in such condition that rat populations are reduced to a minimum.
  4. Rat-proofing of buildings of ports and airports; application of appropriate insecticide with residual effect every 6 months; deratization with effective rodenticide.
  5. International travellers: No country currently requires immunization against plague for entry. Because of the short duration of protection, the recommendation in the face of an existing epidemic or anticipated unusual exposure is for immunization on arrival.

PLEURODYNIA

1. *Identification.*—An acute infectious disease characterized by sudden onset of severe paroxysmal pain commonly localized at the costodiaphragmatic border and accompanied by intermittent fever, headache, anorexia, and malaise. Duration one to three days; remissions frequent. A nonfatal illness usually recognized in localized epidemics. Synonyms: Epidemic Pleurodynia, Bornholm Disease, Epidemic Myalgia, Devil's Grippe.

  Since Coxsackie group B viruses have been repeatedly implicated as causative agents, diagnosis may be aided by isolation from feces and by demonstrating a rise in titer of type-specific neutralizing antibodies in blood serums of early and late illness. Differential count of blood leucocytes is usually normal.

2. *Etiologic agent.*—Various Coxsackie Group B viruses have been implicated. Immunologically distinct Types 1 and 3 have repeatedly been associated with the illness, and other types may occur.

3. *Source and reservoir of infection.*—Coxsackie Group B viruses Types 1 and 3 frequently have been found in feces and also in throat discharges of persons ill with epidemic pleurodynia. These viruses have been found less frequently in well persons in an epidemic area; occasionally, in persons with illnesses not typical of pleurodynia.

4. *Mode of transmission.*—Probably contact with an infected person or with articles freshly soiled with infective material. Group B viruses have been found in sewage, on flies and mosquitoes; the relation to transmission of human disease is not clear.

5. *Incubation period.*—Three to 5 days is usual.

6. *Period of communicability.*—Unknown, but apparently during the acute stage of the disease.

7. *Susceptibility and resistance.*—Susceptibility is probably general, and presumably a type-specific immunity results from infection.

8. *Occurrence.*—The disease is not common; usually occurs in epidemics, with outbreaks reported in Europe, England, Australia, New Zealand, and North America. A summer and early autumn disease, occurring in all age groups but most commonly manifest in children and young adults. Multiple cases frequently occur in a household.

9. *Methods of Control:*

A. Preventive measures: None.

B. Control of the infected individual, contacts, and environment:

1. Report to local health authority: Obligatory report of epidemics; no individual case report, Class 4 (p. 7).
2. Isolation: None.
3. Concurrent disinfection: Prompt and safe disposal of nose and throat discharges and of feces. Articles soiled therewith should be disinfected.
4. Terminal disinfection: None.
5. Quarantine: None.
6. Active immunization: None.
7. Investigation of contacts and source of infection: Of no practical value.
8. Specific treatment: None.

C. Epidemic measures:

1. General notice to physicians of the epidemic occurrence of the disease and the necessity for differential diagnosis of illness which might mistakenly be considered a medical or surgical emergency.

D. International measures: None.

PNEUMONIA

A. Pneumococcal—Acute Lobar Pneumonia

1. *Identification.*—An acute bacterial infection characterized by sudden onset with chill followed by fever, often pain in the chest, usually a productive cough, dyspnea, and leucocytosis. Roentgen-ray examination may disclose pulmonary lesions prior to other evidence of consolidation. Not infrequently pneumococcal pneumonia is bronchial rather than lobar, especially in children, with vomiting and convulsions often the first manifestations. Pneumococcal pneumonia is an important cause of death, generally and among acute infections. The fatality is greatly reduced by antibiotic and chemotherapy; rates formerly were 20 to 40% for hospital patients, but now are ordinarily a small fraction of those figures; much variation according to serologic type of pneumococcus and age of patient, being highest among infants and the aged.

Laboratory confirmation is by bacteriological examination of sputum or discharges of the respiratory tract. A rise in antibody titer between acute-phase and convalescent-phase serums is useful in problem cases, and culture of the blood in severe infections.

2. *Etiologic agent.*—Diplococcus pneumoniae. Pneumococci Types I to XXXII account for about 95% of cases; the remainder are due to rarely recognized types.

3. *Source and reservoir of infection.*—Respiratory tract secretions of patients and carriers. Pneumococci may be found in the upper respiratory tract of healthly members of most communities throughout the world.

4. *Mode of transmission.*—By droplet spread, by direct contact with papatients or carriers, or indirectly through articles freshly soiled with discharges of nose and throat of such persons. Transmission by air-borne particles may be possible but has not been established as important. Person-to-person transmission of the pneumococcus is common, but secondary cases in contacts and attendants are infrequent.

5. *Incubation period.*—Not well determined; believed to be 1 to 3 days.

6. *Period of communicability.*—Unknown; presumably until the discharges of mouth and nose no longer carry the infectious agent in appreciable numbers or in virulent form. Penicillin will eliminate the pneumococcus from most patients within 3 days.

7. *Susceptibility and resistance.*—Resistance is generally high but may be lowered by wet, cold, and exposure, and apparently under certain conditions by physical and mental fatigue and by alcoholism. Inapparent infection is common, particularly with Type 3 pneumococci and strains of higher types. Immunity to the homologous type of pneumococcus usually follows an attack, may last for months or years, and is highly specific. Active immunization against specific types is possible but rarely practical.

8. *Occurrence.*—Common; affecting a large proportion of the population at one time or other between adolescence and old age. No race or color and neither sex is exempt from the disease. More prevalent in industrial cities and lower economic groups. Occurs in all climates and seasons, most often in winter and spring in temperate zones, and in regions where cold, windy, changeable, and inclement weather prevails. Usually sporadic in the United States, but epidemics occur in institutions and in barracks; consistently recurring epidemics have been described in South African mines. A rising incidence is commonly associated with influenza epidemics.

9. *Methods of control:*

  A. Preventive measures:

   1. Whenever practicable and particularly in institutions, barracks, and on shipboard, crowding in living and sleeping places should be avoided. General resistance should be conserved by good food, fresh air, sufficient sleep, temperance in the use of alcoholic beverages, and other hygienic measures.

   2. Chemoprophylaxis with sulfonamide or antibiotic drugs is feasible for closed population groups in time of epidemics, but has not been adequately evaluated.

   3. Active immunization with bacterial vaccines or polysaccharides of prevailing types of pneumococci may be effective for the control of epidemics in limited populations such as mine workers and military units.

  B. Control of the infected individual, contacts, and environment:

   1. Report to local health authority: Obligatory report of epidemics; no individual case report, Class 4 (p. 7). Reported deaths are a better index of frequency of the disease.

     2. Isolation : None.
     3. Concurrent disinfection : Of discharges from nose and throat.
     4. Terminal disinfection : Thorough cleaning and airing.
     5. Quarantine : None.
     6. Immunization : None.
     7. Investigation of contacts and source of infection : Of no practical value.
     8. Specific treatment : Penicillin intramuscularly ; recent reports indicate that oral penicillin G is effective. The tetracycline antibiotics produce comparable results, in event of penicillin sensitivity or delayed response to penicillin. Sulfonamide drugs and erythromycin are usually effective.

   C. Epidemic measures :
     1. Applicable only in outbreaks in institutions or in other limited or closed population groups. General hygienic measures may be supported by immunization against prevailing types of pneumococci or by chemoprophylaxis with sulfonamides or antibiotics.

   D. International measures : None.

B. Bacterial Pneumonia, other than Pneumococcal

1. *Identification.*—An acute febrile disease with pulmonary involvement evidenced by symptoms, physical signs, or Roentgen-ray examination. Often occurs in association with other infections of the respiratory tract, particularly epidemic influenza. The fatality with adequate treatment is low but appreciable, and variable according to infectious agent and age of the patient.

     Appropriate bacteriologic examination of sputum, nasopharyngeal swabs and blood aid materially in diagnosis.

2. *Etiologic agents.*—Various pathogenic bacteria of the mouth, nose, and throat, as Streptococcus pyogenes or Group A hemolytic streptococci, Staphylococcus aureus, Klebsiella pneumoniae (Friedlander's bacillus) and Hemophilus influenzae.

3. *Source and reservoir of infection.*—Discharges from mouth and nose of patients and carriers.

4. *Mode of transmission.*—By droplet spread, by direct contact with patient or carrier or indirectly through articles freshly soiled with discharges of nose or throat of such persons.

5. *Incubation period.*—Variable, usually short, 1 to 3 days.

6. *Period of communicability.*—Unknown ; probably while the infectious agent is present in discharges of nose and throat of patients. For many of the agents involved, antibiotic therapy greatly decreases the period of communicability.

7. *Susceptibility and resistance.*—Susceptibility appears to be low grade ; highest in infants and young children, and in the aged. Immunity varies with the infecting organism and is probably minimal except for type-specific immunity to Group A streptococci. Immunization procedures are not feasible.

8. *Occurrence.*—Worldwide in distribution and a frequent disease in infancy and old age, and in winter months in temperate climates. No racial selectivity. Usually sporadic, but epidemics occur in association with influenza, measles or other respiratory infection.

9. *Methods of control:*

    A. Preventive measures:

        1. Good personal hygiene; avoid crowding in institutions and hospitals.

        2. Immunization against Influenza (p. 91) and chemoprophylaxis of Streptococcal Infections (p. 170) may be applied to limited or general populations.

    B. Control of the infected individual, contacts, and environment:

        1. Report to local health authority: Obligatory report of epidemics; no individual case report, Class 4 (p. 7).
Identification of a preceding respiratory infection is of public health significance.

        2. Isolation: None.

        3. Concurrent disinfection: Of discharges from mouth and nose and of articles soiled therewith.

        4. Terminal disinfection: Thorough cleaning and airing.

        5. Quarantine: None.

        6. Immunization: None.

        7. Investigation of contacts and source of infection: Of no practical value.

        8. Specific treatment: Streptococcal: Same as pneumococcal pneumonia. Staphylococcal: Procaine penicillin; if organism proves resistant, tetracycline antibiotics as in pneumococcal pneumonia; sensitivity tests with the organism isolated may aid in selecting the most suitable antibiotic. H. influenzae: The tetracyclines and chloramphenicol are all effective; combined sulfadiazine-streptomycin is also used. K. pneumoniae: (Friedlander's) Streptomycin initially, then the tetracyclines or chloramphenicol after the acute phase.

    C. Epidemic measures:

        1. Applicable only in outbreaks in institutions or in other limited or closed population groups when associated with influenza, measles or other respiratory infection. Active immunization against influenza and passive immunization of infants and children against measles may be employed. Chemoprophylaxis may be effective but has not been adequately evaluated.

    D. International measures: None.

C. Primary Atypical Pneumonia (Virus Pneumonia)

1. *Identification.*—An acute respiratory infection characterized by gradual and insidious onset, constitutional symptoms of chilliness, feverishness, headache, malaise and fatigue, and respiratory symptoms of cough and expectoration. Initial physical signs in lungs are minimal but develop later. Early patchy infiltration, demonstrable by roentgenographic examination of chest, is often more extensive than clinical findings suggest. Count and distribution of leucocytes usually normal. Duration of illness averages about a week and complications are infrequent; the fatality is about 1 per 1,000.

    Development of cold hemagglutinins during convalescence or of agglutinins for streptococcus MG, or both, confirms diagnosis in one-half to two-thirds of cases.

Differentiation required from psittacosis, influenza, Q fever, and a number of other infections with similar clinical manifestations.

2. *Etiologic agent.*—Most cases apparently due to a virus or viruses, not yet isolated or characterized or given specific name.

3. *Source and reservoir of infection.*—Probably discharges from mouth and nose of patients, and of persons with mild, unrecognized infections.

4. *Mode of transmission.*—By intimate contact with a patient or with articles freshly soiled with discharges of nose and throat of such person.

5. *Incubation period.*—Believed to be 7 to 21 days, commonly 12.

6. *Period of communicability.*—Unknown; presumably during late incubation and throughout febrile illness.

7. *Susceptibility and resistance.*—The low incidence in general populations and low attack rate among contacts suggest a relatively high resistance. Most infected persons suffer no more than mild respiratory illness with no pneumonia. Degree and duration of immunity after attack are unknown; second attacks are rare. No available immunization.

8. *Occurrence.*—World-wide distribution, as a sporadic, endemic, and occasionally epidemic disease especially in institutions and military populations. No reliable attack rates for civilian populations; rates of 10 per 1000 per annum are recorded among military populations. Incidence greatest during winter months in temperate zones, with much variation from year to year and in different geographic areas. No selectivity for race or sex. Occurs at all ages, but recognized disease is more frequent among adolescents and young adults.

9. *Methods of control:*

A. Preventive measures:

1. When possible, crowding in living and sleeping quarters should be avoided, especially in institutions, in barracks, and on shipboard. General resistance should be maintained by adequate food, sufficient sleep, fresh air, and good personal hygiene.

B. Control of the infected individual, contacts, and environment:

1. Report to local health authority: Obligatory report of epidemics; no individual case report, Class 4 (p. 7).
2. Isolation: None.
3. Concurrent disinfection: Of discharges from nose and throat.
4. Terminal disinfection: Thorough cleaning and airing.
5. Quarantine: None.
6. Immunization: None.
7. Investigation of contacts and source of infection: Of no practical value.
8. Specific treatment: Beneficial results in individual cases have been reported through use of tetracycline antibiotics. Symptomatic and supportive treatment is effective in most instances.

C. Epidemic measures:

No certainly effective measures for control are available. Isolation precautions in epidemic situations may be helpful.

D. International measures: None.

POLIOMYELITIS

1. *Identification.*—An acute illness, usually febrile, varying in early symptomatology, but usually with headache and almost always a characteristic stiffness of neck and spine and tightness of hamstring muscles, often justifying an examination of spinal fluid. In about half such cases a lower neurone paralysis develops within the first few days of illness, with a marked tendency for spontaneous improvement after reaching its height. If the patient is first seen after the acute stage has passed, diagnosis depends upon detection of a flaccid paralysis irregularly involving various muscles or muscle groups. Presumptive diagnosis in nonparalytic cases depends upon detection of clinical manifestations compatible with the illness and demonstration of moderate increase in cells or protein in the spinal fluid. A form of illness presumptively poliomyelitis (abortive) but with only vague symptoms and without signs referable to the central nervous system, occurs during epidemics. Inapparent infections exceed clinical cases at least several hundred-fold. Fatality rates vary from 4 to 15%, for bulbar poliomyelitis from 5 to 60%. Synonym: Infantile Paralysis.

   Virus may be isolated from feces or throat secretions; rising titer of antibodies to one type of virus can be demonstrated by complement fixation or neutralization test. Microscopic and chemical examination of spinal fluid is useful in excluding other diseases.

2. *Etiologic agent.*—Poliomyelitis viruses, Types 1, 2 and 3, readily distinguished immunologically, although having minor common antigenic components.

3. *Source of infection.*—Pharyngeal secretions and feces of infected persons, most frequently those not suffering from clinically recognizable disease, especially children.

4. *Mode of transmission.*—By direct contact and droplet spread through close association with infected persons. In rare instances milk has been a vehicle. Flies and sewage have been found contaminated with virus, but no reliable evidence establishes insects, water, food other than milk, or sewage in transmission of the infection.

5. *Incubation period.*—From 7 to 21 days, commonly 12.

6. *Period of communicability.*—Greatest communicability is apparently in late incubation and first few days of acute illness, virus usually being present in throat and feces; persists in feces for 3 to 6 weeks or more.

7. *Susceptibility and resistance.*—Susceptibility to infection is general, but few develop paralytic disease. Type specific immunity is acquired by infection, whether clinically apparent or inapparent, and probably is of long duration; second attacks are rare and may be due to infection by virus of another type. Infants born of immune mothers have a transient passive immunity.

8. *Occurrence.*—Infection prevails throughout most of the world; occurs both sporadically and in epidemics at irregular intervals, with the highest incidence in summer and early fall. Paralytic disease is more frequent in temperate zones. Wide variations in incidence occur from year to year and region to region. Even during epidemics the incidence of paralytic cases in large cities has rarely exceeded 100 per 100,000 population. Outbreaks in smaller com-

munities tend to reach this level more frequently, and occasionally to be much higher. In the United States during the past decade the reported incidence of poliomyelitis has ranged from 7 to 37 cases per 100,000 population; approximately half of reported cases are non-paralytic. Children from one to 16 years of age are more frequently attacked than adults. In several countries, including the United States, older children and young adults constitute a higher proportion of reported cases than formerly. In congested areas of the tropics and subtropics, inapparent infection with all three types of virus is usual during the first few years of life, and paralytic disease is infrequent among older children and adults.

9. *Methods of control:*

A. Preventive measures: None other than those of 9B.

B. Control of the infected individual, contacts and environment:

1. Report to local health authority: Obligatory case report in most states and countries, Class 2A (p. 7). Individual cases should be specified as paralytic or nonparalytic.

2. Isolation: For one week from date of onset, or for the duration of fever if longer.

3. Concurrent disinfection: Of throat discharges and feces and of articles soiled therewith.

4. Terminal disinfection: None.

5. Quarantine: Of unproved value. While quarantine of family contacts is theoretically worthwhile, there is no evidence of practical benefit because of the large number of unrecognized infections in the community.

6. Immunization: None; gamma globulin of no practical value.

7. Investigation of contacts and source of infection: Thorough search for sick persons, especially children, to locate unrecognized and unreported cases.

8. Specific treatment: None; attention to prevention and management of paralysis.

C. Epidemic measures:

1. General notice to physicians of prevalence or increased incidence of the disease, description of usual character of onset and necessity for diagnosis and medical care, particularly for bed rest of patient.

2. Isolation in bed of all children with fever, pending diagnosis.

3. Education in such technics of bedside nursing as will prevent tranmission of infectious discharges from patients isolated at home.

4. Protection of children so far as practicable against unnecessary close contact with other persons, especially with other family groups or outsiders during epidemic prevalence of the disease. Urban schools should not be closed nor opening delayed, but intensive or competitive athletic programs should be postponed. Rural schools, particularly where buses are used to gather children from sparsely populated areas, and boarding schools which draw children from areas free of the disease and at a distance, should not be opened until the epidemic is clearly declining.

5. Postponement of elective nose or throat operations.

6. Avoidance by children of excessive physical strain as in violent exercise during an epidemic or with known exposure.

7. Postponement of inoculation of any precipitated type antigen of children over 6 months of age if the slightly increased risk of poliomyelitis is considered greater than the risk of disease for which immunization is intended.

8. Avoidance of unnecessary travel and visiting, especially of children, during high prevalence of infection.

9. Gamma globulin has been used as a means for general passive immunization in communities where incidence is high. The protective capacity is controversial, the conditions for its use undefined, and the theoretical indications difficult to meet; of no practical value. Vaccines for active immunization are in experimental use.

D. International measures: Telegraphic notification of epidemics by national health authorities to WHO.

PSITTACOSIS

1 *Identification.*—An acute generalized viral infection having an onset with fever and headache; early pneumonic involvement; cough initially absent or non-productive, later usually present and productive; sputum light yellow and extremely viscous; anorexia extreme; constipation the rule; pulse usually slow in relation to temperature; great prostration; delirium common; relapses not uncommon. Fatality is from 5 to 40% for reported cases; mild atypical infections not infrequent. Normal or slightly increased numbers of leucocytes early, leucopenia later. Synonym: Ornithosis.

Laboratory diagnosis during first week of illness is by inoculation of mice with sputum or blood; repeated trials are often necessary. A rise in titer of complement fixing antibodies may be demonstrated; serums from lymphogranuloma venereum infection also react.

2. *Etiologic agent.*—The viruses of psittacosis or ornithosis, antigenically related to that of lymphogranuloma venereum.

3. *Source and reservoir of infection.*—Infected parrots, parakeets, love birds, canaries, pigeons, ducks, turkeys, chickens and other birds. Apparently healthy birds occasionally transmit infection through virus in cloacal discharges. Sputum from infected persons is an occasional source. Mammalian hosts, calves and sheep, have been identified but their relation to disease of man is not determined.

4. *Mode of transmission.*—Contact with infected birds or their recent surroundings, chiefly household pets but also infected pigeons in cities; occasionally through a human infection. Virus may be airborne; laboratory infection frequent.

5. *Incubation period.*—In human infections, 6 to 15 days.

6. *Period of communicability.*—During acute severe illness, especially when coughing. Birds characteristically have latent infection but at irregular intervals appear sick and shed virus in large quantities.

7. *Susceptibility and resistance.*—All ages susceptible, but more severe among older adults; one attack usually confers immunity.

8. *Occurrence.*—Usually in sudden familial outbreaks among persons exposed to sick or apparently healthy birds. Deaths mainly confined to persons older than 30 years. An occupational infection in pet shops, aviaries and poultry processing plants.

9. *Methods of control:*

 A. Preventive measures:

  1. Strict regulation of import or traffic in birds of parrot family based on quarantine and laboratory examination.

  2. Quarantine of pet shops known to have harbored infected birds, until thoroughly cleaned.

  3. Education of community in the danger of making house pets of birds of the parrot family, particularly birds recently imported or with likely history of contact with sick birds.

 B. Control of the infected individual, contacts and environment:

  1. Report to local health authority: Obligatory case report in most states and countries, Class 2A (p. 7).

  2. Isolation: Important during febrile acute stages. Nurses caring for patients with a cough should wear adequate gauze masks.

  3. Concurrent disinfection: Of all discharges.

  4. Terminal disinfection: Thorough wet cleaning and exposure to sunlight.

  5. Quarantine: Buildings having housed birds should not be used by humans until thoroughly cleaned and disinfected.

  6. Immunization: None.

  7. Investigation of contacts and source of infection: Trace source of suspect birds. Infected birds should be killed and bodies immersed in 2 percent cresol. While feathers are wet, spleen, liver and kidneys should be aseptically removed, frozen in sterile container, and sent to nearest available laboratory. Carcasses should be burned after autopsy.

  8. Specific treatment: The tetracycline antibiotics (aureomycin and terramycin) and chloramphenicol continued several days after temperature becomes normal.

 C. Epidemic measures: See 9B7.

 D. International measures: Reciprocal respect for national regulations designed to control importation of psittacine birds by land, water, or air.

Q FEVER

1. *Identification.*—Q fever is characterized by sudden onset, chilly sensations, headache, weakness, malaise, severe sweats, and considerable variation in severity and duration. Pneumonia, similar to that of atypical pneumonia, occurs in the majority of cases as well as mild cough, scanty expectoration, chest pain, minimal physical findings, and little or no upper respiratory involvement. Chronic general infections have been reported. The fatality before introduction of specific therapy was not more than 1%; it is now negligible.

Laboratory diagnosis is by complement fixation reaction through demonstration of rise in antibody titer between acute and convalescent specimens; by agglutination test; or by recovery of the causative organism from blood of the patient, readily accomplished but hazardous to laboratory workers.

2. *Etiologic agent.*—Rickettsia burneti (Coxiella burneti).

3. *Source and reservoir of infection.*—Milk of infected domestic animals and dust-laden air of barns and pens; carcasses of infected mammals, bodies of patients dead of the disease, and contaminated wool, straw and laundry have caused outbreaks. Ticks, wild animals (bandicoots), cattle, sheep and goats serve as natural reservoirs.

4. *Mode of transmission.*—Commonly by air-borne dissemination of rickettsiae; milk from infected cows may be responsible for some cases since commercial pasteurization reduces but may not eliminate viable R. burneti; also direct contact with meat from infected animals.

5. *Incubation period.*—Usually 2 to 3 weeks.

6. *Period of communicability.*—Communicability from man to man has not been demonstrated.

7. *Susceptibility and resistance.*—Susceptibility is general. An attack confers immunity of unknown duration. Vaccination increases resistance.

8. *Occurrence.*—Reported from all continents except South America. Endemic in California where infection exists enzootically in animals raised for meat and milk; has occurred in explosive epidemics in a number of areas in United States, among workers in diagnostic laboratories, stock yards, meat packing and rendering plants and wool processing factories. The largest outbreaks were among troops of World War II in Italy and Greece.

9. *Methods of control:*

A. Preventive measures:
   1. Immunization with inactivated vaccine prepared from R. burneti infected yolk sac appears so useful in protecting laboratory workers that it should be considered for others in hazardous occupations.
   2. Pasteurization preferably above 62.9° C. (145° F.), or boiling of milk from cows, goats and sheep.

B. Control of the infected individual, contacts, and environment:
   1. Report to local health authority: Obligatory case report in most states and countries, Class 2B (p. 7). Value limited by need for special laboratory aid in diagnosis.
   2. Isolation: None.
   3. Concurrent disinfection: Of sputum and blood, and articles freshly soiled therewith.
   4. Terminal disinfection: None.
   5. Quarantine: None.
   6. Immunization: Of case contacts, unnecessary.
   7. Investigation of contacts and source of infection: Search for history of contact with cattle, sheep and goats, consumption of raw milk, or direct or indirect association with a laboratory handling R. burneti.
   8. Specific treatment: The tetracycline antibiotics or chloramphenicol, administered orally and continued for several days after afebrile; reinstitute if relapse occurs.

C. *Epidemic measures*: Individual outbreaks are generally of short duration; control measures are essentially limited to observation of exposed persons and therapy for those ill. In hyperendemic situations immunization should be considered for persons at greatest risk.

D. *International measures*: Control of importation of domestic animals.

RABIES

1 *Identification.*—An invariably fatal acute encephalitis that begins with a sense of apprehension, headache, fever, malaise and indefinite sensory changes often referred to the point of inoculation. The disease progresses to paresis or paralysis; spasm of muscles of deglutition on attempt to drink. Delirium and convulsions follow, ending in death from respiratory paralysis. Duration from onset to death varies from 2 to 6 days. Synonym: Hydrophobia.

Verification of diagnosis depends upon demonstration of Negri bodies in nerve cells of the brain or upon animal inoculation.

2. *Etiologic agent.*—The virus of rabies.

3. *Source and reservoir of infection.*—The source of infection is the saliva of rabid animals. Reservoirs include any of a large group of wild and domestic Canidae, including the dog, fox, coyote, wolf, and also cat, skunk, raccoon, opossum and other biting mammals. Vampire and fruit eating bats are infected in South and Central America; infection of insectivorous bats recently recognized in the United States.

4. *Mode of transmission.*—By bite of a rabid animal or on rare occasions contact of saliva of such animals with a scratch or other break in the skin.

5. *Incubation period.*—Usually 2 to 6 weeks or longer; depends on extent of laceration, site of wound in relation to richness of nerve supply, and length of nerve path to brain.

6. *Period of communicability.*—In the dog, for 3 to 5 days before onset of clinical symptoms and through the clinical course of the disease; rarely communicated from man to man.

7. *Susceptibility and resistance.*—Susceptibility general among mammals. Natural immunity is unknown in man or among animals subject to rabies. Prophylactic antirabic treatment of infected humans ordinarily will prevent the disease if begun soon after injury and if the wound does not extensively involve the distribution of the facial nerve. Antirabic vaccination leads to artificial active immunity in dogs.

8. *Occurrence.*—Uncommon in man; primarily a disease of animals. Occurs throughout the world except in Australia, New Zealand, Hawaii and other Pacific Islands, some of the West Indies, Great Britain and the Scandinavian peninsula. Urban rabies is a problem of dogs and occasionally other pets; sylvatic or rural rabies primarily of wild biting animals, with sporadic infection of dogs and domestic livestock.

9. *Methods of control:*

A. Preventive measures:

1. Detention and observation for 10 days of dogs and other animals suspected of rabies or having bitten a person. Rabid animals have a change in behavior, excitability or paralysis, and death occurs within 10 days.

2. Immediate destruction or 6 months detention of dogs or cats bitten by known rabid animals.

3. Emphasis on preventive vaccination of dogs; all owned dogs in congested areas should be kept on leash when not within homes of owners. Ownerless dogs should be destroyed by public authority.

4. Education of the public and especially of dog owners and police in handling suspected rabid dogs or those that have bitten a person. Such dogs should be confined for 10 days and observed for symptoms of rabies; should not be killed until rabies is established clinically; the intact head should then be submitted for laboratory examination.

5. Cooperative programs with wild life and conservation authorities toward reduction of foxes and other reservoir animals in areas of sylvatic rabies.

B. Control of the infected individual, contacts and environment:

1. Report to local health authority: Obligatory case report required in most states and countries, Class 2A (p. 7).

2. Isolation: Through duration of illness; immediate attendants should be warned of the hazard of inoculation through saliva of patient.

3. Concurrent disinfection: Of saliva and articles soiled therewith.

4. Terminal disinfection: None.

5. Quarantine: None.

6. Immunization: Human anti-rabies vaccination is based on the following principles:

a. When apprehended, observe animal for 10 days. Give vaccine during this 10 day period to persons with severe bites on head or hands, especially with known rabies in the area. Give vaccine if laboratory diagnosis of rabies is established in the animal. In less severe bites, give vaccine if animal develops clinical rabies or dies during observation, whether or not laboratory diagnosis is established.

b. If animal is not apprehended, vaccine should be administered when rabies is known to be present in the area. If vaccine is administered, 14 consecutive daily doses are usual. In severe exposures, vaccine is given daily for 21 days. Due to recognized occurrence of post-vaccinal paralysis, vaccine should not be given unless the skin is broken. Chances that rabies will develop must carefully be weighed against the small but finite chance of paralysis. For persons who have previously received anti-rabic vaccine, particularly within one year, consideration should be given to reducing the schedule of inoculations. Anti-rabies serum is useful in severe exposures in conjunction with vaccination.

7. Investigation of contacts and source of infection: Search for rabid animal and for persons and other animals bitten.
8. Specific treatment: For clinical rabies, none. Wounds caused by bite or scratch of an animal with rabies or suspected rabies are thoroughly cleaned and irrigated with a solution of tincture of green soap, or other antiseptic detergent; corrosive agents such as fuming nitric acid are not recommended.

C. Epidemic measures:
1. Establishment of area control under authority of state laws, regulations and local ordinances, in cooperation with appropriate wildlife, conservation and livestock sanitary authorities.
2. Strict enforcement of regulations requiring leashing of owned dogs, and of collection, detention and destruction of ownerless, stray or unvaccinated dogs found off owner's premises.
3. Widespread vaccination of dogs, preferably with an attenuated live vaccine.
4. Education of the public in the necessity of complying with restrictions on dogs, of vaccinating dogs, of seeking immediate medical attention if bitten by a dog, of confining and observing animals that inflict bites, of prompt reporting to the police of dogs manifesting strange behavior, and of reporting rabies in dogs and dog bites to the local health authority.

D. International measures: Strict compliance by common carriers and by travellers with national laws and regulations that institute quarantine or require vaccination of dogs intended for introduction into rabies-free areas.

RAT–BITE FEVER

Two diseases are included under the general term of rat-bite fever; one, also known as Haverhill fever, is caused by Streptobacillus moniliformis; the other, also known as Sodoku, is caused by Spirillum minus. The first disease has priority in recognition and description. Because of similarity in clinical and epidemiological behavior, and because Streptobacillus moniliformis infection is more common in the United States, only it is presented in detail. The essential variations manifested by Spirillum minus infection are noted under that disease.

A. Streptobacillus Moniliformis Infection

1. *Identification.*—Usually a history of rat bite within 10 days; primary edematous lesion; swelling of regional lymph nodes; sharp febrile paroxysms often alternating with afebrile intervals, and accompanied by a morbilliform and petechial rash, polyarthritis, and leucocytosis. Ulceration of the primary lesion may occur; also regional lymphadenitis. Fatality may reach 10% in untreated cases. Synonym: Haverhill Fever.

Bacteriologic examination of primary lesion, lymph nodes, blood and joint fluids, or serum test by specific agglutination, or mouse inoculation. Caution should be exercised lest the experimental mouse or rat be already naturally infected.

2. *Etiologic agent.*—Streptobacillus moniliformis (Streptothrix muris rattis, Haverhillia multiformis, Actinomyces muris).

3. *Source and reservoir of infection.*—An infected rat, rarely other rodents (squirrel, weasel). Sporadic cases without reference to bite have been recorded.

4. *Mode of transmission.*—By the bite of an infected animal; animal blood escapes from the injured or diseased buccal mucosa into the wound, or the conjunctival secretion of the rat may contaminate the wound. Blood from an experimental laboratory animal may infect man. Localized epidemics may occur from contaminated milk or milk products (Haverhill fever); the means of contamination is not known, whether through infection of cows by rat bite, or direct contamination of milk by rats.

5. *Incubation period.*—Three to 10 days, rarely longer.

6. *Communicability.*—Not known to be transmitted from man to man.

7. *Susceptibility and resistance.*—No data for man.

8. *Occurrence.*—Distribution is world-wide. Uncommon in North and South America and in most European countries; case reports, however, show this to be the usual form of rat-bite fever in the United States.

9. *Methods of control:*

   A. Preventive measures:
   1. Reduction of rat population. Rat proofing of dwellings.
   2. Pasteurization of milk may help in preventing Haverhill fever.

   B. Control of the infected individual, contacts, and environment:
   1. Report to local health authority. Obligatory report of epidemics; no individual case report, Class 4 (p. 7).
   2. Isolation: None.
   3. Concurrent disinfection: None.
   4. Terminal disinfection: None.
   5. Quarantine: None.
   6. Immunization: None.
   7. Investigation of contacts and source of infection: Not practicable.
   8. Specific treatment: Penicillin; tetracycline antibiotics may be substituted. Treatment should be continued for seven to 10 days.

   C. Epidemic measures: Grouped cases presenting the typical symptoms require search for epidemiologic evidence of a relation to milk supply.

   D. International measures: None.

B. Spirillum Minus Infection

A sporadic rat-bite fever, Sodoku, is caused by Spirillum minus (Spirocheta morsus muris). It is less frequently observed in the United States than Streptobacillus moniliformis infection, but in Japan and the Far East is reported to be the common form. The incidence of rat-bite fever appears to be greater there than in western countries, although the data are inadequate. The fatality rate is approximately 10%. Clinically, Spirillum minus infection differs from streptobacillus infection in the usual absence of arthritic symptoms, and a more plaque-like rash. The incubation period is generally longer, one to 3 weeks, and usually more than 7 days. Laboratory methods are essential for differentiation of the two diseases.

RELAPSING FEVER

Two disease entities, having minor clinical variations and distinguishable principally by differences in mode of transmission and geographic distribution, are known as relapsing fever. One is louse-borne, the other tick-borne.

A. Louse-Borne Relapsing Fever

1. *Identification.*—An epidemic spirochetal disease with short febrile paroxysms lasting 2 or 3 days, alternating with afebrile periods of 3 or 4 days and resulting in 2 to 10 relapses, more commonly the lesser number; each attack terminates by crisis and the average duration of the disease is 13 to 16 days. Transitory petechial-like rashes are common during the initial fever. The fatality ranges between 2 and 10%.

    Diagnosis is through demonstrating the infectious agent in dark-field preparations of fresh blood, stained thick blood films, or by intraperitoneal inoculation of white rats with 15 to 25 cc. of blood taken during the pyrexial period and before crisis.

2. *Etiologic agent.*—Borrelia recurrentis, a spirochete. Numerous specific names have been given to morphologically identical but biologically different spirochetes isolated from cases of relapsing fever in widely separated endemic areas.

3. *Source and reservoir of infection.*—Immediate source is infected louse; reservoir is blood of infected persons. Inter-epidemic reservoir is unknown.

4. *Mode of transmission.*—By crushing an infected louse, Pediculus humanus, into the bite-wound or into an abrasion of the skin.

5. *Incubation period.*—Up to 12 days, average 7 days.

6. *Period of communicability.*—Not communicable from man to man. The louse becomes infective 4 to 5 days after ingestion of blood from an infected person and remains so for life (20 to 40 days).

7. *Susceptibility and resistance.*—Susceptibility is general. The duration of immunity after clinical attack is unknown but probably does not exceed two years.

8. *Occurrence.*—In limited localities in Europe and among peoples of Asia, North and South Africa, and Central America who are louse infested. Epidemics are commonly incidental to war and famine or other situations where malnourished, over-crowded populations with poor personal hygiene favor multiplication and wide dissemination of the vector. Not reported in the United States for many years.

9. *Methods of control:*

A. Preventive measures:

1. Routine application of insecticide with residual effect, such as DDT or a number of other compounds, at appropriate intervals to populations living under conditions favoring the development of lousiness.

2. Individual prophylaxis through application of insecticide, DDT or equivalent, at appropriate intervals to clothing as dusting powder or by impregnation.

3. Improvement of living conditions with provision for frequent bathing and washing of clothing.

B. Control of the infected individual, contacts, and environment:

1. Report to local health authority: Case report universally required by international regulation, Class 1 (p. 6).

2. Isolation: After proper chemical delousing of patient, clothing and bedroom, and of patient's household contacts, isolation is not required.

3. Concurrent disinfection: None.

4. Terminal disinfection: Careful terminal application of insecticides to body and clothing of patient where death occurs before this has been done.

5. Quarantine: Exposed lousy susceptibles are quarantined for 15 days or may be released after application of insecticide with residual effect, for example DDT.

6. Immunization: None.

7. Investigation of contacts and source of infection: For the individual case, unprofitable; a community effort (see 9C).

8. Specific treatment: Penicillin G in adequate dosage; tetracyclines and chloramphenicol are also effective. Patients with central nervous system involvement, particularly with inadequate dosage, will likely experience relapse. Arsenical therapy, neo-arsphenamine and mapharsen, is widely used.

C. Epidemic measures:

1. The most important measure for the rapid control of relapsing fever, where reporting has been good and the number of cases small, is application of insecticides with residual effect to contacts of all reported cases. Where infection is known to be widespread, systematic application of residual insecticide to all persons in the community is indicated; 2–5% DDT in an inert powder, talc or pyrophyllite for dusting.

D. International measures:

1. Telegraphic notification of WHO and of adjacent countries, by governments, of the existence of an epidemic of relapsing fever. An internationally quarantinable disease.

2. Measures applicable to ships, aircraft and land transport arriving from relapsing fever areas are specified in International Sanitary Regulations (WHO Techn. Rep. Ser. No. 41, Geneva, 1951).

B. Tick-Borne Relapsing Fever

1. *Identification.*—Regularly an endemic disease with a clinical course similar to that of louse-borne infection, except that relapses are more frequent, averaging 6 or 7; deaths are rare. A satisfactory history of tick bite is unlikely and evidence of bite is seldom found.

   Diagnosis is by demonstrating the infectious agent in thick smears of blood at time of febrile attack, or from blood of mice, rats or monkeys inoculated with patient's blood at that time.

2. *Etiologic agent.*—Borrelia duttoni, a spirochete. Numerous specific names have been given to morphologically identical but biologically different spirochetes isolated from cases of relapsing fever in widely separated endemic areas.

3. *Source and reservoir of infection.*—Immediate source, infected tick; reservoir, wild rodents.

4. *Mode of transmission.*—Man is infected by the bite or coxal fluid of an infected tick, principally one of five species of the genus Ornithodoros; in the United States, O. turicata and O. hermsi; O. rudis and O. talaje are vectors in Central and South America; O. moubata in tropical Africa; and O. tholozani in Near East, Middle East, and Far East. Transovarian infection occurs in ticks.

5. *Incubation period.*—Three to 6 days, but may be as short as 2 days or as long as 12.

6. *Period of communicability.*—Not communicable from man to man. Ticks can live for years without feeding and remain infective.

7. *Susceptibility and resistance.*—Susceptibility is general. The duration of immunity after recovery is indefinite, but probably not more than 2 years.

8. *Occurrence.*—Widespread throughout tropical Africa. Foci have been observed in Spain, North Africa, Arabia, Iran, India, and parts of Central Asia as well as in North and South America. In the United States human cases of tick-borne relapsing fever have been found in limited localities of 13 western states.

9. *Methods of control:*

   A. Preventive measures:

      1. Avoidance of tick-infested caves, camp sites, shacks, and ground areas. Exposed persons should use tick repellent on exposed areas of skin, such as dimethylphthalate, indalone, Rutgers 612, or a number of other compounds now under investigation. Clothing may be impregnated with repellent by sprayers or by dipping. Lindane can be used as a residual spray in buildings. The habits of argasid ticks differ from those of Ixodidae and consequently pose a different problem in prevention. Ticks of this genus attack, rapidly engorge, and promptly leave the body of the host.

   B. Control of the infected individual, contacts, and environment:

      1. Report to local health authority: In selected endemic areas (USA); in many countries not a reportable disease, Class 3B (p. 7).
      2. Isolation: None.
      3. Concurrent disinfection: None.
      4. Terminal disinfection: None.
      5. Quarantine: None.

6. *Immunization*: None.
7. *Investigation of contacts and source of infection*: Important.
8. *Specific treatment*: See Treatment of Louse-borne Relapsing Fever, p. 145.

C. Epidemic measures: Reduction of tick population in living quarters by periodic dusting with insecticides.

D. International measures: None.

RHEUMATIC FEVER

1. *Identification.*—Rheumatic fever appears as an occasional sequella of Group A hemolytic streptococcal upper respiratory infection, and sometimes in the absence of such recognized prior infection. The main clinical manifestations are migratory polyarthritis, carditis, chorea, subcutaneous nodules and erythema marginatum. Fever, rapid pulse, non-traumatic epistaxis, abdominal and precordial pain, pallor, anorexia, weight loss, a fast sedimentation rate, leuocytosis and electrocardiographic changes are a second group of findings of lesser diagnostic significance. With a history of previous attack, combinations of the above suggest recurrence of rheumatic fever. Mild and inapparent infections occur, their relative frequency unknown; definite and even severe right heart disease develops in absence of evident acute rheumatic fever. A leading cause of death among children of the United States, aged 6 to 10 years; the fatality is appreciable, commonly 3 to 5% in endemic areas. Synonym: Acute Articular Rheumatism.

   Bacteriologic or serologic (chiefly antistreptolysin O) evidence of a preceding Group A streptococcal infection adds diagnostic weight to suggestive symptoms.

2. *Etiologic agent.*—Unknown. Attacks are usually precipitated by Group A streptococcal respiratory infections, frequently unrecognized or so mild as to have had no medical attention.

3. *Source and reservoir of infection.*—Unknown.

4. *Mode of transmission.*—Unknown.

5. *Incubation period.*—Not applicable. Symptoms appear about 2 to 3 weeks after a recognized Group A streptococcal infection.

6. *Period of communicability.*—Not known to be communicable; the preceding streptococcal infection which may precipitate rheumatic fever is communicable but usually has subsided by the time rheumatic fever develops.

7. *Susceptibility and resistance.*—All age groups are susceptible; the greatest incidence is in children from 6 to 12 years of age. The disease has a natural tendency to recur; no evidence that immunity develops.

8. *Occurrence.*—A frequent disease in temperate zones throughout the world; in the United States most prevalent in Rocky Mountain region, New England, and North and Central Atlantic states; lowest in the South and Southwest. Seasonal incidence is that of streptococcal infections, in the United States a peak during spring months and a low point during summer and early autumn. Reliable data on frequency in tropical areas are not available; the impression of a lesser prevalence than in temperate zones is not always supported.

Predilection for race or sex has not been defined. For unknown reasons, incidence and mortality of rheumatic fever are declining.

9. *Methods of control:*

A. Preventive measures:

1. No practical measures of prevention except those for Group A streptococcal infections (see Scarlet Fever, p. 170).

B. Control of the infected individual, contacts and environment:

1. Report to local health authority: In selected endemic areas (USA); in many states and countries not a reportable disease, Class 3B (p. 7). Areas of high incidence will profit materially by encouraging individual case report over prescribed periods sufficient to acquire epidemiological data necessary for improved methods of control.

2. Isolation: None.

3. Concurrent disinfection: None.

4. Terminal disinfection: None.

5. Quarantine: None.

6. Immunization: None.

7. Investigation of contacts and source of infection: None.

8. Specific treatment: Individuals known to have had rheumatic fever or convalescent from that disease should receive chemoprophylaxis for long periods thereafter, possibly throughout life, at least until age 18 years, and past that age for a period of 5 years from last attack. Either a sulfonamide drug or penicillin may be employed, given orally throughout the year. Prior to prophylaxis, proper treatment should be instituted to free the patient of Group A streptococci (see Scarlet Fever, p. 171).

Salicylates are the method of choice in management of the acute phase, preferably acetylsalicylic acid, also sodium salicylate, continued for duration of active disease. Patients must be protected from intercurrent infection, particularly Group A hemolytic streptococci.

C. Epidemic measures: Epidemics of rheumatic fever occur only in association with epidemics of Group A streptococcal infections. Proper therapy of the streptococcal infection (see Scarlet Fever) will prevent the subsequent development of rheumatic fever and thus prevent about half of the cases of rheumatic fever.

D. International measures: None.

RICKETTSIALPOX

1. *Identification.*—Rickettsialpox is characterized by an initial skin lesion, chills, fever, varicelliform rash, and a mild to severe course; even before specific therapy, case fatality was less than 1%. The initial lesion appears as a firm red papule about a week in advance of fever, most commonly on the covered parts of the body, the papule becomes vesicular, then covered by a scab and after about 3 weeks leaves a small pigmented scar. Fever, often preceded by chills, is remittent with peaks of 39.4° C. to 40.6° C. (103° F. to 105° F.), usually lasting less than one week. Headache, muscular pain, and general malaise are frequent. The secondary rash is manifest 3 to

4 days after onset of fever; has no characteristic distribution but seldom occurs on palms or soles; progresses through papular and papulovesicular stages, lasting usually less than one week and leaving no scars; local lymphadenopathy occurs in the region of the initial lesion, but splenomegaly or generalized lymph node enlargement is uncommon.

Specific diagnosis is by complement fixation test, positive between the second and third week of the disease. Sera from patients with rickettsialpox give Weil-Felix reactions with proteus OX antigens below the level regarded as significant in other rickettsial diseases.

2. *Etiologic agent.*—Rickettsia akari, a member of the spotted fever group of rickettsiae.

3. *Source and reservoir of infection.*—Infected house mice (Mus musculus musculus).

4. *Mode of transmission.*—From mouse to mouse and probably from mouse to man by a rodent mite, Allodermanyssus sanguineus.

5. *Incubation period.*—Probably 10 to 24 days.

6. *Period of communicability.*—Not communicable from man to man. Duration of infectivity of mouse for mite, and mite for mouse or man are unknown.

7. *Susceptibility and resistance.*—Susceptibility appears general. Duration of immunity after attack is unknown.

8. *Occurrence.*—Approximately 150 cases occur annually in New York City, principally among inhabitants of apartment houses where the mouse, mite and rickettsia maintain a natural cycle of infection. A few cases have been recognized in Boston, Hartford, and Philadelphia; occurrence in other areas is probable.

9. *Methods of control:*

A. Preventive measures:

   1. Rodent and mite control by elimination of mice and mouse harborages, including proper care and firing of incinerators in dwellings, and application of residual miticides (aldrin and others) to infested areas. Commercial vaccine not available and not currently needed.

B. Control of the infected individual, contacts and environment:

   1. Report to local health authority: In selected endemic areas (USA); in most states and countries not a reportable disease, Class 3B (p. 7).
   2. Isolation: None.
   3. Concurrent disinfection: None.
   4. Terminal disinfection: None.
   5. Quarantine: None.
   6. Immunization: None.
   7. Investigation of contacts and source of infection: Search for infested mice in dwelling and, if feasible, undertake isolation of rickettsiae from rodents and mites.
   8. Specific treatment: The tetracycline antibiotics and chloramphenicol are equally effective.

C. Epidemic measures: When groups of cases occur in the same or adjacent dwellings the preventive measures listed under 9A should be applied. Other inhabitants should be observed and promptly treated if the disease develops.

D. International measures: None.

RIFT VALLEY FEVER

1. *Identification.*—An acute viral infection, primarily of sheep and other animals, which develops in man with unusual suddenness, a fever of 38.2° C. to 40.5° C. (101° F. to 105° F.) lasting for several days, and has a course resembling that of dengue. Relapse is so common as to suggest a two-stage disease. A wide variety of clinical manifestations includes headache, rigors, backache, vertigo, muscle and joint pain, tenderness of the eyeballs, photophobia, epistaxis, and prostration. Leucopenia is a characteristic feature. The illness lasts for a week to 10 days with much prostration; convalescence is ordinarily rapid and death is rare, in contrast to the disease in sheep, especially lambs, which is highly fatal. Synonym: Enzootic Hepatitis.

   Laboratory confirmation is by isolation of virus from blood through mouse inoculation; specific neutralizing antibodies are demonstrable in convalescence.

2. *Etiologic agent.*—The virus of Rift Valley fever.

3. *Source and reservoir of infection.*—Sheep, cattle, and goats are reservoirs of infection for man. An unidentified wild animal is conceived as the primary reservoir.

4. *Mode of transmission.*—Indefinite; probably through bite of an infected mosquito or other blood sucking arthropod. The mechanism of transmission in laboratory infections is unknown. Numerous cases in man relate to persons performing autopsies on sheep or laboratory animals, housewives preparing meat, and to milk.

5. *Incubation period.*—Usually 5 to 6 days.

6. *Period of communicability.*—During viremia of animals and man; in man, first 3 days of the disease. Mosquitoes become infectious after about 20 days; believed to remain infective through life.

7. *Susceptibility and resistance.*—Man is relatively resistant in comparison with sheep. Neutralizing antibodies have been demonstrated years after recovery from laboratory infection.

8. *Occurrence.*—An uncommon and sporadic disease of man; as a naturally acquired infection reported only in Africa, from the Union of South Africa north to the Anglo-Egyptian and French Sudan. Epizootics occur among sheep; cattle and goats are sporadically infected.

9. *Methods of control:*

   A. Preventive measures:

      1. Precautions in care and handling of infected animals, and their products.

      2. Protection against mosquitoes and other possible arthropod vectors in endemic areas.

      3. The frequency of laboratory accidents is such as to require extreme care by those working with the virus.

   B. Control of the infected individual, contacts and environment:

      1. Report to local health authority: In selected endemic areas; not a reportable disease in most countries, Class 3B (p. 7).

      2. Isolation: None.

      3. Concurrent disinfection: None.

      4. Terminal disinfection: None.

150

5. Quarantine : None.
6. Immunization : None.
7. Investigation of contacts and source of infection : Within the immediate premises, of little value. A community problem, see 9C.
8. Specific treatment : None.

C. Epidemic measures : Not applicable to man ; a sporadic disease. The problem is of domestic animals and the surrounding biologic environment. The need is for epidemiologic investigation in attempt to identify arthropod vector and natural reservoir.

D. International measures : None.

RINGWORM

Ringworm is a general term applied to mycotic infections of keratinized areas of the body (hair, skin and nails). Various genera and species of a group of fungi known collectively as the dermatophytes are causative agents. For convenience in presentation, the dermatomycoses are subdivided according to sites of infection as follows : Tinea capitis (ringworm of the scalp), tinea corporis (ringworm of the body), tinea pedis (athlete's foot) and tinea unguium (ringworm of the nails). Synonyms : Favus, Jockey-Itch, Athlete's Foot, The Dermatomycoses.

A. Ringworm of Scalp (Tinea Capitis)

1 *Identification.*—Infection begins as a small papule and spreads peripherally, leaving scaly patches of alopecia (baldness). Infected hairs become brittle and break off easily. Occasionally boggy, raised and suppurative lesions develop, called kerions. Examination of the scalp under Wood light for fluorescence is helpful in certain ringworm infections.

Microscopic examination of hairs, cleared with sodium hydroxide solution, shows spores within the hair (endothrix type) or surrounding it (ectothrix type). The fungus should be cultured for genus and species identification.

Favus of the scalp is a variety of tinea capitis, caused by Trichophyton schoenleini and characterized by formation of small, yellowish, cup-like crusts or scutulae giving the appearance of being stuck on to the scalp. Affected hairs do not break off but become gray and lusterless, eventually fall out and leave baldness which may be permanent. Microscopic examination of the hair in sodium hydroxide shows no spores, but the interior of the hair is filled with long branching mycelial filaments and characteristic air spaces.

Tinea capitis is distinguished easily from piedra, a fungus infection of the hair occurring in South America and some countries of Southeast Asia, an infection characterized by hard "gritty" nodules in the hair shafts.

2. *Etiologic agent.*—Various species of Microsporum and Trichophyton. Identification of genus and species is important epidemiologically and for estimation of prognosis.

3. *Source and reservoir of infection.*—Sources are such materials as barber clippers, toilet articles or clothing contaminated with infected hair. Reservoirs are scalp lesions of man or lesions of infected animals, especially dogs, cats and cattle.

4. *Mode of transmission.*—Direct contact with sources or reservoirs of infection.

5. *Incubation period.*—10 to 14 days.

6. *Period of communicability.*—As long as infected lesions are present, and as long as viable spores are present on contaminated materials.

7. *Susceptibility and resistance.*—Children before the age of puberty are notoriously susceptible to Microsporum infections and most adults are resistant. All ages are subject to Trichophyton infections but children are more susceptible. No immunity is developed.

8. *Occurrence.*—Ringworm of the scalp caused by Microsporum audouini is widespread in the United States, particularly in urban areas. M. canis infection occurs both in rural and urban areas wherever infected cats and dogs are present. Trichophyton mentagrophytes and T. verrucosum (faviforme) infections are common in rural areas in association with infected cattle and horses. T. tonsurans infections are epidemic in urban areas in Southwestern United States and Mexico. Incidence in children is higher than adults, males are infected more frequently than females; significant differences in race have not been noted. Infection of animals is more common in damp cold seasons, especially when confined to barns, and incidence of human infection with animal-transmitted strains is thus higher in colder weather.

9. Methods of control:

   A. Preventive measures: In epidemic areas young children should be surveyed by Wood light before entering school. The public, especially parents, should be warned of the dangers of acquiring infection from other infected children as well as from dogs, cats and other animals. Effective control of animal ringworm.

   B. Control of the infected individual, contacts and environment:
      1. Report to local health authority: Obligatory report of epidemics; no individual case report, Class 4 (p. 7).
         School outbreaks should be reported to school authorities.
      2. Isolation: Impractical. The patient should be under a regulated regime of treatment with periodic visits to physician or clinic. Hair should be covered with a cap which can be sterilized frequently.
      3. Concurrent disinfection: Contaminated caps should be boiled after use.
      4. Terminal disinfection: None.
      5. Quarantine: Not practicable.
      6. Immunization: None.
      7. Investigation of contacts and source of infection: Household contacts, and pets and farm animals, for evidence of infection.
      8. Specific treatment: Ointments containing salicylanilid, copper undecylenate or any one of a variety of similar compounds. Epilation by Roentgen-ray is instituted if progress is not satisfactory. Examine weekly and take cultures to assure recovery is complete.

C. Epidemic measures: Epidemics in a school or institution require special measures such as education of children and parents, and enlistment of services of doctors and nurses for diagnosis. Follow-up surveys are important.

D. International measures: Examination of scalps of immigrants coming from areas of high prevalence of favus or T. tonsurans or T. violaceum infections. Infected persons should be detained, placed under treatment and entry deferred until free of the disease, a procedure not to be loosely applied to all ringworm infection.

B. Ringworm of Body (Tinea Corporis)

1. *Identification.*—Cutaneous infections other than of the scalp, bearded areas and feet, characteristically appearing as flat spreading ring-shaped lesions. The periphery is reddish, vesicular or pustular, and may be dry and scaly or moist and crusted. As lesions progress peripherally, the central area often clears and skin appears normal.
   Scrapings from the advancing margins, cleared in sodium hydroxide and examined microscopically, show segmented branching filaments. Final identification is by culture.

2. *Etiologic agent.*—Epidermophyton floccosum and various species of Microsporum and Trichophyton.

3. *Source and reservoir of infection.*—Sources are contaminated floors, shower stalls, benches and similar articles; reservoir is skin lesions of man.

4. *Mode of transmission.*—Direct contact with sources or reservoirs of infection.

5. *Incubation period.*—10 to 14 days.

6. *Period of communicability.*—As long as viable spores are present on contaminated materials.

7. *Susceptibility and resistance.*—Susceptibility is general. Clinical manifestations are commonly exaggerated under conditions of friction and excessive perspiration, as in axillary and inguinal regions.

8. *Occurrence.*—World-wide and relatively frequent. Males are infected more than females. All ages are susceptible and racial differences are immaterial.

9. *Methods of control:*

   A. Preventive measures: Adequate sterilization of towels and general cleanliness in showers and dressing rooms of gymnasiums, especially repeated washing of benches. A fungicidal agent such as cresol should be used for disinfection.

   B. Control of the infected individual, contacts and environment:
      1. Report to local health authority: Obligatory report of epidemics; no individual case report, Class 4 (p. 7).
         Case report to school authority of infections of children, involving exposed parts of the body is desirable.
      2. Isolation: Infected children should be excluded from gymnasiums, swimming pools and activities likely to lead to exposure of others.
      3. Concurrent disinfection: Of clothing in contact with infected parts of the body.
      4. Terminal disinfection: None.

    5. Quarantine: None.

    6. Immunization: None.

    7. Investigation of contacts and source of infection: Examination of school and household contacts, and of household pets and farm animals.

    8. Specific treatment: Thorough bathing with soap and water, removal of scabs and crusts, and application of any of a number of ointments containing salicylic acid or one of the higher fatty acids (propionic acid, undecylenic acid).

  C. Epidemic measures: Education of children and of parents concerning the nature of the infection, its mode of spread and necessity of maintaining good body hygiene.

  D. International measures: None.

C. Ringworm of Foot (Tinea Pedis)

1. *Identification.*—Scaling or cracking of the skin, especially between the toes, or blisters containing a thin watery fluid are so characteristic that most laymen recognize "athlete's foot." In severe cases, vesicular lesions appear on various parts of the body, especially the hands. These dermatophytids do not contain the fungus and represent an allergic reaction to fungus products.

    Microscopic examination of sodium hydroxide-treated scrapings from lesions between the toes reveals segmented branching filaments.

2. *Etiologic agent.*—Epidermophyton floccosum and various species of Microsporum and Trichophyton.

3. *Source and reservoir of infection.*—Sources of infection are infected persons or contaminated floors, shower stalls and other articles used by them. Reservoir is skin lesions of infected persons.

4. *Mode of transmission.*—Direct contact with sources or reservoirs of infection.

5. *Incubation period.*—Approximately 10 to 14 days.

6. *Period of communicability.*—As long as infected lesions are present and as long as viable spores are present on contaminated materials.

7. *Susceptibility and resistance.*—Susceptibility is variable and infection may be inapparent. Second attack is frequent.

8. *Occurrence.*—World-wide and a common disease. Adults more often affected than children; males more than females. No differences in racial susceptibility. Infections are more prevalent in hot weather.

9. *Methods of control:*

  A. Preventive measures:

    1. As for tinea corporis above.

    2. Maintenance of strict personal hygiene, with special care in drying areas between toes after bathing.

  B. Control of the infected individual, contacts and environment:

    1. Report to local health authority: Official report not ordinarily justifiable, Class 5 (p. 7). School outbreaks should be reported to school authorities.

    2. Isolation: None.

3. Concurrent disinfection : Socks from heavily infected individuals should be boiled to prevent reinfection. Shoes should be placed in a box and subjected to formaldehyde for several hours, followed by airing to prevent irritation of skin from residual formalin.
4. Terminal disinfection : None.
5. Quarantine : None.
6. Immunization : None.
7. Investigation of contacts and source of infection : None.
8. Specific treatment : Ointments, as recommended for tinea corporis, may be used. Exposure of feet to air through wearing sandals is often beneficial.

C. Epidemic measures : Thorough cleaning and washing down of gymnasiums, showers, and similar sources of infection. Education of the public concerning the nature of the infection and its mode of spread.

D. International measures : None.

D. Ringworm of Nails (Tinea Unguium)

1. *Identification.*—A chronic infection involving one or more nails of the hand or foot. The nail gradually thickens, becomes discolored and brittle, and an accumulation of caseous-appearing material forms beneath the nail.

   Microscopic examination of sodium hydroxide preparations of the nail and of detritus beneath the nail shows segmented branching mycelial filaments. The diagnosis should be confirmed by culture.

2. *Etiologic agent.*—Epidermophyton floccosum and various species of Trichophyton.

3. *Source and reservoir of infection.*—Source is presumably direct extension from infections of foot, possibly contaminated floors and shower stalls ; reservoir is skin or nail lesions of infected persons.

4. *Mode of transmission.*—Unknown.

5. *Incubation period.*—Unknown.

6. *Period of communicability.*—As long as infected lesions are present.

7. *Susceptibility and resistance.*—Unknown ; injury to nail predisposes to infection.

8. *Occurrence.*—Common. Adult males more frequently infected than females. No seasonal or racial differences.

9. *Methods of control :*

   A. Preventive measures : The measures described above for prevention of tinea pedis.

   B. Control of the infected individual, contacts and environment :
   1. Report to local health authority : Official report not ordinarily justifiable, Class 5 (p. 7).
   2. Items 2 through 7, see tinea pedis above.
   8. Specific treatment : Scrape off as much of affected nail as possible. Apply ointments or other medication of types described for tinea pedis. Repeat frequently until nail appears normal.

   C. Epidemic measures : Not applicable.

ROCKY MOUNTAIN SPOTTED FEVER

1. *Identification.*—This prototype of the diseases caused by the spotted fever group of rickettsiae is an infectious endangiitis characterized by sudden onset of fever, ordinarily persisting for two weeks, headache, conjunctival injection and a maculopapular rash. The rash appears on the extremities about the third day and spreads rapidly to most of the body, including palms and soles, before becoming petechial. The fatality is about 20% in absence of specific therapy; death is uncommon with prompt treatment.

   The Weil-Felix reaction with Proteus OX-19 and usually with OX-2 becomes positive late in the second week, complement fixation tests, using specific rickettsial antigen, a few days later.

2. *Etiologic agent.*—Rickettsia rickettsii.

3. *Source and reservoir of infection.*—Infected ticks. In eastern and southern United States the common vector is the dog tick, Dermacentor variabilis; in northwestern United States, the wood tick, Dermacentor andersoni; in southwestern United States occasionally the Lone Star tick, Amblyomma americanum. In Brazil, Amblyomma cajennense is the common vector. The rabbit tick Haemaphysalis leporis palustris is infected in nature but does not bite man. The infection is passed from generation to generation in ticks and probably is maintained by infected and non-infected larvae feeding upon susceptible wild rodents.

4. *Mode of transmission.*—Ordinarily by bite of infected tick but contamination of skin with crushed infected tick tissues or feces may lead to infection in man.

5. *Incubation period.*—From 3 to about 10 days.

6. *Period of communicability.*—Not directly communicable in nature from man to man.

7. *Susceptibility and resistance.*—Susceptibility is general. One attack confers immunity which may or may not be permanent. Suitable vaccines induce immunity artificially.

8. *Occurrence.*—Throughout most of the United States during spring and summer but most prevalent in Rocky Mountain and Middle Atlantic seaboard states. In western United States, adult males are most affected while in the East children are more frequently attacked; infection rates are related to opportunity for contact with infected ticks, and fatality rates increase with age. Infection also occurs in western Canada, western and central Mexico, Colombia and Brazil. Although limited to the Western Hemisphere, the disease is closely related to tick-borne rickettsial infections of other continents.

9 *Methods of control:*

   A. Preventive measures:

   1. Personal prophylaxis by avoiding tick-infested areas when feasible, by careful removal of ticks from the person as promptly as possible without crushing and with protection of the hands when removing ticks from animals. Some of the newer insect repellents (n-n-butyl-acetanilide) are of value against ticks.

2. Measures for reducing tick populations are generally impractical. Clearing the land, reducing small wild mammal populations, stray dog control and removing ticks from livestock by dipping may help. In selected areas direct application of appropriate insecticides effects excellent control of some tick vectors. DDT is used; newer preparations to include lindane, aldrin and others are undergoing field trial.

3. Vaccines containing killed R. rickettsii lessen the chance of infection and lower case fatality. Since advent of specific therapy, vaccination is generally limited to persons at high risk. Reinforcing doses at yearly intervals are necessary to maintain protection.

B. Control of the infected individual, contacts, and environment:

1. Report to local health authority: In selected endemic areas (USA); in many countries not a reportable disease, Class 3B (p. 7).

2. Isolation: None.

3. Concurrent disinfection: All ticks on patients should be destroyed.

4. Terminal disinfection: None.

5. Quarantine: None.

6. Immunization: Of case contacts, unnecessary.

7. Investigation of contacts and source of infection: Not profitable except as a community measure; see 9C.

8. Specific treatment: The tetracycline antibiotics or chloramphenicol in daily oral doses until patient is afebrile (usually 3 days) and for one or two additional days.

C. Epidemic measures: In hyperendemic areas particular attention should be paid to identification of infected ticks and infested areas, and to recommendations in 9A1, 2.

D. International measures: None.

RUBELLA

1. *Identification.*—A mild febrile infection with a rash of variable character, sometimes resembling that of measles, sometimes that of scarlet fever, and sometimes an admixture of both; few or no constitutional symptoms but almost always enlargement of the postauricular, sub-occipital or post-cervical group of lymph nodes; occasionally others. Mild catarrhal symptoms may be present; absence of Koplik spots differentiates the disease from measles. Infection without a rash has been produced experimentally. Leucopenia is usual during fever. Synonym: German Measles.

Roseola infantum (exanthem subitum) is to be distinguished from rubella by clinical and epidemiologic differences, notably the onset of rash after subsidence of fever and predilection for infants rather than older children and adults.

2. *Etiologic agent.*—The virus of rubella.

3. *Source and reservoir of infection.*—Nasopharyngeal secretions of infected persons; viremia shortly before and after onset of symptoms.

4. *Mode of transmission.*—By droplet spread or direct contact with patient, or by indirect contact with articles freshly soiled with discharges from nose or throat. Airborne transmission also occurs.

5. *Incubation period.*—From 14 to 21 days; usually 18 days.

6. *Period of communicability.*—For at least 4 days after onset of catarrhal symptoms and probably not much longer, the exact period being undetermined. Highly communicable.

7. *Susceptibility and resistance.*—Susceptibility is general among young children. An attack usually confers permanent immunity.

8. *Occurrence.*—Epidemic in expression, mostly in childhood, but with more adult patients than in measles; more prevalent in winter and spring than in other seasons. World wide in distribution and a common communicable disease.

9. *Methods of control.*—Efforts to control rubella are prompted by the hazard of congenital defects in offspring of women who acquire the disease during pregnancy. The extent of the risk is indefinite, but approximately 10 to 20% of living infants born after maternal rubella during the first trimester of pregnancy have anomalies.

A. Preventive measures:

   1. No attempt should be made to protect female children in good health against exposure to the disease before puberty.

B. Control of the infected individual, contacts and environment:

   1. Report to local health authority: Obligatory report of epidemics; case report ordinarily serves no useful purpose; may be required specifically where contacts include susceptible women in first 4 months of pregnancy, Class 4 (p. 7).

   2. Isolation: None, except where contacts include a woman in early pregnancy; then under direction of the attending physician for 5 days after onset.

   3. Concurrent disinfection: None.

   4. Terminal disinfection: None.

   5. Quarantine: None.

   6. Immunization: Immune serum globulin (gamma globulin) appears to have some value in passive protection against rubella; results conflicting. Until evidence to the contrary and because of the serious risk to offspring, may be administered to adult female contacts with no definite history of rubella and exposure within the first 4 months of pregnancy; other non-immune family contacts may be included.

   7. Investigation of contacts and source of infection: Of no practical value except to clarify possible confusion with scarlet fever; and to identify adult female contacts in the first 4 months of pregnancy.

   8. Specific treatment: None.

C. Epidemic measures: No procedures in common use can be relied upon as a means of effective control of the disease or of epidemics.

D. International measures: None.

SCABIES

1. *Identification.*—An infection of the skin caused by the itch mite and characterized by itching, by burrows which appear as slightly elevated grayish white lines and house the mite with eggs, and by papules and vesicles. The latter often become pustular from secondary infection by scratching. Lesions are most prominent in folds of the skin such as finger webs, elbow creases, armpits, between the thighs, and under the breasts of women; no fatality. Synonym: The Itch.

   The itch mite is identified by hand lens in scrapings from the burrows, the eggs microscopically.

2. *Etiologic agent.*—Sarcoptes scabiei, the itch mite.

3. *Source and reservoir of infection.*—Persons harboring the itch mite.

4. *Mode of transmission.*—Transfer of young female mite by direct contact with the skin of infected persons; to a limited extent, by underclothing and linen recently used by infected individuals.

5. *Incubation period.*—Several hours are required for the itch mite to dig a burrow and become implanted. Itching and subsequent lesions may develop in 24 to 48 hours, or may be delayed for a week or two.

6. *Period of communicability.*—Until itch mites and eggs are destroyed, a period that varies from 1 to 2 weeks depending on treatment used.

7. *Susceptibility and resistance.*—Anyone may become infected or reinfected. Initial infection results in sensitization accompanied by a rather marked tissue reaction and followed by a decreased susceptibility to reinfection.

8. *Occurrence.*—Widespread and independent of climate, sex, or race. Commonly associated with overcrowding, body uncleanliness, neglect and lack of soap and water. Single infections in a family, without spread to others of the group, are uncommon. Epidemics occur characteristically in barracks, camps, and institutions.

9. *Methods of control:*

   A. Preventive measures:

      1. Cleanliness of body, underclothing and bed covering. Attention to proper laundering of linen.

   B. Control of the infected individual, contacts and environment:

      1. Report to local health authority: Official report not ordinarily justifiable; presence in schools should be reported to school authorities, Class 5 (p. 7).
      2. Isolation: Children should be excluded from school until adequately treated. Infected persons should be denied common recreation and bathing facilities.
      3. Concurrent disinfection: Proper laundering of underwear and personal linen.
      4. Terminal disinfection: Unnecessary if effective treatment has been carried out.
      5. Quarantine: None.
      6. Immunization: None.
      7. Investigation of contacts and source of infection: Search for unreported or unrecognized cases in companions or in other members of the household.

8. Specific treatment: (a) Benzyl benzoate; a 25% emulsion is applied with a wide, flat brush to the entire body, giving attention to areas with many lesions. A second application is made within 24 hours, and at 48 hours a bath is taken. (b) Hexachlorocyclohexane (kwell); a 1% ointment is rubbed into the skin avoiding the eyes. A second application may be necessary. The drug is toxic in high concentration or if used repeatedly. (c) Sulfur; a 5% sulfur ointment is applied to the skin and repeated in 24 and 48 hours. The same underwear should be worn during this period. After another 24 hours a bath is taken.

C. Epidemic measures:
  1. Segregation of infected individuals.
  2. Provision of convenient facilities for prompt treatment of the infection.
  3. Encouragement of bodily cleanliness and use of clean underclothes and bedding by people living in crowded quarters.
D. International measures: None.

SCHISTOSOMIASIS

1. *Identification.*—A blood-fluke (trematode) disease in which the adult male and female worms live in veins of the host (mainly mesenteric, portal and pelvic). Eggs there deposited produce minute granulomata and scars in organs in which they lodge. Early manifestations are remittent fever, giant urticaria, abdominal discomfort, right upper quadrant tenderness, and eosinophilia which may reach 85%; accompanied or soon followed by blood in feces or urine. Late manifestations are cirrhosis of liver with ascites and splenomegaly, or severe chronic cystitis or other pelvic manifestations. Eggs may be deposited in spinal cord or brain with resulting neurological manifestations. Death is uncommon except from complications, but more frequent for S. japonicum than for other species. Synonym: Bilharziasis.

    Definitive diagnosis is by finding the characteristic eggs in feces or urine; light infections require special concentration methods or rectal biopsy.

2. *Etiologic agents.*—Schistosoma mansoni, S. haematobium and S. japonicum.

    The larvae of certain other schistosomes of birds and rodents may penetrate the human skin causing a dermatitis known as "swimmer's itch." These schistosomes do not mature in man.

3. *Source and reservoir of infection.*—Immediate source is snails infected with larval forms. Reservoir is usually persons harboring the infection. Pigs, cattle, water buffalo and dogs, also field mice and wild rats, are animal hosts of S. japonicum.

4. *Mode of transmission.*—The eggs of S. haematobium leave the body mainly with the urine; those of S. mansoni and S. japonicum with the feces. The egg hatches in water and the liberated larva or miracidium enters a suitable fresh water snail host. Free swimming larvae, cercariae, emerge from the snail after several weeks

and penetrate the human skin, usually while the person is swimming or wading; they enter the blood stream, are carried to blood vessels of the liver, develop to maturity, and then migrate to veins of the abdominal cavity. Adults of S. mansoni and S. japonicum usually remain in mesenteric veins; those of S. haematobium usually migrate through anastomoses into the pelvic veins. Eggs are deposited in venules and, by necrosis of tissue, escape into the lumen of bowel or bladder, but may lodge in other organs.

5. *Incubation period.*—Systemic manifestations usually begin when the worms are reaching maturity, about 4 to 6 weeks after infection. Eggs usually are found in feces or urine a week or two after onset of symptoms.

6. *Period of communicability.*—As long as eggs are discharged in urine or feces of infected persons which may be 25 years or longer. Infected snails may give off cercariae for several months.

7. *Susceptibility and resistance.*—Susceptibility is general; whether or not resistance develops as a result of infection is controversial.

8. *Occurrence.*—S. mansoni occurs in the West Indies, northeastern and eastern South America, the Arabian peninsula, and Africa. S. haematobium occurs in Africa and in parts of the Middle East. S. japonicum occurs in the Orient (Japan, China, Formosa, Philippines, Celebes). No species is indigenous to continental North America. In some endemic areas more than half of the population is infected.

"Swimmer's itch" is prevalent among bathers in lakes in many parts of the world including North America; also in certain coastal sea water beaches.

9. *Methods of control:*

   A. Preventive measures:
   1. Disposal of feces and urine so that eggs will not reach bodies of fresh water containing snail intermediate host. Control of animals infected with S. japonicum.
   2. Treatment of snail breeding places with molluscacides, and other methods of snail destruction.
   3. Provision of water for drinking, bathing and washing clothes from sources free from cercariae.
   4. Provision of cercaria-repellent or cercaria-proof clothing for persons required to enter contaminated water.
   5. Education of people in endemic areas regarding mode of transmission and methods of protection.
   6. Mass treatment of infected persons in endemic areas may help to reduce transmission but in the past has not materially reduced incidence.

   B. Control of the infected individual, contacts and environment:
   1. Report to local health authority: In selected endemic areas; in many countries not a reportable disease, Class 3C (p. 7).
   2. Isolation: None.
   3. Concurrent disinfection: Sanitary disposal of feces and urine.
   4. Terminal disinfection: None.
   5. Quarantine: None.
   6. Immunization: None.

7. Investigation of contacts and source of infection: Examine contacts for infection from a common source. The search for the source is a community effort, see 9C.

8. Specific treatment: For S. mansoni and S. haematobium, fuadin intramuscularly. For S. haematobium, nilodin, miracil dihydrochloride, is efficacious in light infections, less so in heavy infections; disagreeable side effects but no serious toxicity. For S. japonicum, tartar emetic intravenously; toxic side-effects occur.

C. Epidemic measures: In areas of high incidence, or in endemic areas where non-indigenous groups such as military forces become infected, snail breeding places should be carefully determined and treated with molluscacides; entering infected water should be prohibited. Clean water should be provided, population should be examined for infection, and infected persons treated.

D. International measures: None.

SCRUB TYPHUS

1. *Identification.*—A rickettsial disease transmitted by trombiculid mites and characterized by a primary lesion and a rash late in the first week of fever. The primary lesion, usually on a protected area of skin and representing the site of attachment of the infected mite, precedes the acute febrile onset by several days. Headache, conjunctival injection and lymphadenopathy accompany the fever. A dull red maculopapular eruption appears on the trunk, extends to the extremities, and disappears in a few days. Cough and roentgenographic evidence of pneumonitis are common. In the absence of specific antibiotic therapy, fever lasts for 14 days. The fatality in untreated cases varies with locality (1 to 40%) and is regularly higher in older age groups. Synonyms: Tsutsugamushi Disease, Mite-borne Typhus.

Isolation of the etiologic agent in mice, and specific complement fixation tests supplement the Weil-Felix reaction (Proteus OXK) in laboratory diagnosis of the disease.

2. *Etiologic agent.*—Rickettsia tsutsugamushi.

3. *Source and reservoir of infection.*—Infected larval mites of Trombicula akamushi and related species which vary with locality, are the source of infection; reservoir, wild rodents. The nymphs and adults do not feed on vertebrate hosts. The agent is passed from generation to generation in mites; also maintained by a mite-wild rodent-mite cycle.

4. *Mode of transmission.*—By the bite of infected mites.

5. *Incubation period.*—Usually 10 to 12 days but varies from 6 to 21.

6. *Period of communicability.*—Not communicable from man to man.

7. *Susceptibility and resistance.*—Susceptibility is general. An attack confers prolonged immunity against the homologous strain of R. tsutsugamushi but only transient immunity against heterologous strains. Heterologous infection within a few months results in mild disease but such infection after a year produces the typical

illness. Second and even third attacks of naturally acquired scrub typhus are not uncommon in persons who spend their lives in endemic areas. Inactivated vaccine is useless as an immunizing agent.

8. *Occurrence.*—Scrub typhus occurs in eastern and southeastern Asia, northern Australia, the Indian subcontinent and adjacent islands. It is a place disease acquired by man in one of the innumerable small sharply delimited "typhus islands" where the rickettsiae, the vector and the rodent reservoir exist simultaneously. Occupational habits greatly influence sex distribution, but with few exceptions the disease is restricted to adult workers who frequent scrub or overgrown terrain. In the Pescadores Islands children are more often attacked because infected rodents and mites inhabit rock walls around gardens of homes. Epidemics occur when susceptibles are brought into endemic areas, a repeated observation among troops of World War II; in certain regiments and battalions 20 to 50% of men were infected within weeks or months.

9. *Methods of control:*

   A. Preventive measures:
      1. The aim is to prevent contact with infected mites, to eliminate mites and rodents from particular sites and to promote resistance to the disease.
      2. Personal prophylaxis against the mite vector is by use of clothes and blankets impregnated with miticidal chemicals, together with application of mite repellents to exposed skin surfaces.
      3. In military practice selected camp sites are cleared of vegetation by stripping with a bulldozer, the vegetation destroyed by burning, the area sprayed with residual miticidal chemicals (effective for several weeks or a month), and rodent control measures instituted.
      4. Attempts to render man insusceptible to scrub typhus are generally impractical. That result can be attained in special instances by chemoprophylaxis with chloramphenicol, or immunization by a combined procedure of infection with living unattenuated vaccine and suppression of clinical disease by chemoprophylaxis.

   B. Control of the infected individual, contacts and environment:
      1. Report to local health authority: In selected endemic areas, with clear distinction from endemic and epidemic typhus; in many countries not a reportable disease, Class 3A (p. 7).
      2. Isolation: None.
      3. Concurrent disinfection: None.
      4. Terminal disinfection: None.
      5. Quarantine: None.
      6. Immunization: None.
      7. Investigation of contacts and source of infection: None.
      8. Specific treatment: One of the tetracycline antibiotics or chloramphenicol orally in a loading dose followed by divided doses daily until patient is afebrile (average 30 hours). If treatment is instituted within the first three days a second course should be given about the 8th day after onset to prevent relapse.

C. Epidemic measures:
1. Rigorously employed procedures described in 9A2 and 9A3 for all persons in the affected area.
2. Daily observation for fever and appearance of primary lesion of all persons at risk; institute treatment promptly at first indication of illness.
3. Consider use of chemoprophylaxis for key personnel in area; combined live vaccine-chemoprophylaxis may be considered prior to entering areas of known risk.

D. International measures: None.

SMALLPOX

1. *Identification.*—An exanthematous disease characterized by sudden onset with fever, chills, headache, severe backache and prostration, continuing for 3 to 4 days. The temperature then falls and a rash appears which passes through stages of macule, papule, vesicle and pustule, forms crusts and finally scabs which fall off at about the end of the third week. The eruption is usually symmetrical and general, more profuse on prominences, extensor surfaces and surfaces exposed to irritation than on protected surfaces, flexures and depressions. Most abundant and earliest on the face, next on forearms, wrists and hands, and favoring the limbs, especially distally, more than the trunk. More abundant on shoulders and chest than on loins or abdomen, but lesions may be so few as to be overlooked.

Smallpox varies from a mild disease (variola minor) with a fatality under one percent to a severe condition (classical smallpox, variola major) with about 30 percent fatality; in recent years the disease has kept closely to these extremes, breeding true to type as regards severity. An uncommon fulminating form, hemorrhagic smallpox, is characterized by purpura, hemorrhages into the skin, and death within 3 to 4 days, usually before the typical rash appears. The mild type, variola minor or alastrim, has mild prodromal symptoms, a discrete and scanty rash and a more rapid progression of lesions. Previous vaccination commonly leads to modification of both the mild and classical forms of the disease, in timing and maturation of rash, and in other clinical features.

Laboratory confirmation can be had within 24 hours through demonstration of specific antigen in vesicular and pustular fluid from cutaneous lesions by complement-fixation with rabbit antivaccinal serum; or within a few days through isolation of smallpox virus from chick embryos inoculated with such materials.

2. *Etiologic agent.*—The virus of smallpox.

3. *Source and reservoir of infection.*—Lesions of skin and mucous membrane and respiratory discharges of patients.

4. *Mode of transmission.*—By contact with persons sick with the disease. Contact need not be intimate; aerial transmission may occur over short distances within closed spaces. Also spread by articles or persons freshly contaminated by respiratory discharges or by lesions of the skin and mucous membranes of the sick; scabs remain infectious for variable periods.

5. *Incubation period.*—Seven to 16 days, commonly 12 days. A good working rule in epidemiological investigations is 10 days from rash to onset of second illness, or 14 days from rash to rash, the latter being the more useful in field practice.

6. *Period of communicability.*—From first symptoms to disappearance of all scabs and crusts, a period of about 2 to 3 weeks. Most communicable in the early stages of the disease.

7. *Susceptibility and resistance.*—Susceptibility is universal, although exposure of a susceptible person does not always result in the disease. Permanent immunity usually follows recovery; second attacks are rare. Immunity acquired by vaccination gradually diminishes; it may be completely effective for less than 2 years or for more than 20 years.

8. *Occurrence.*—Distributions within countries of the world range from sporadic to endemic to epidemic, varying widely according to immunity status of a population and frequency of imported infection. Incidence is greatest in winter and least in summer. The disease is still a serious problem in parts of Asia, Africa and South America.

9. *Methods of control:*

A. Preventive measures:

1. Vaccination at about the third month of age, revaccination on entering school, and of all persons facing unusual exposure, as in travel to endemic regions or presence of smallpox. Revaccination under conditions of sustained high risk may be practiced at intervals as short as every six months, as with troops in military operations.

2. Measures to assure available supplies of potent glycerinated smallpox vaccine maintained below freezing up to the hour of vaccination, to include time in transit or shipment. Dried calf lymph vaccine is available for use under special conditions, mainly tropical.

3. To avoid complications, insertion of vaccine should be over a small area of skin, not over one-eighth inch in any direction, and preferably by multiple pressure method or by acupuncture. If the scratch method is employed, care should be taken to avoid drawing blood. The site should be kept dry and cool without the use of shields or dressings. The deltoid area of the arm is the preferred site; leg vaccination should be avoided. Primary vaccination should be about the third month of age, provided the child has no eczema or other contraindication; patients with eczema should not come in contact with recently vaccinated persons. Vaccination during the warmer months is preferably avoided.

Revaccination with a fully potent vaccine, of persons immunized more than ten years previously, gives at least 50% of vaccinoid (accelerated) reactions. The site of revaccination should be carefully observed and the reaction recorded twice, on the 3rd and 9th days after vaccination, to determine whether the maximum diameter of redness occurred under three days (immediate or early reaction, formerly called immune reaction), or after 7 days (vaccinia), or intermediate between the two (vaccinoid reaction). The common result is either an immediate or accelerated reaction. The accelerated reaction indicates persisting protection; the immediate reaction, if marked by a firm indurated papule at the site of revaccination, probably does. Errors in interpretation of the early reaction are frequent; inactive vaccine sometimes gives the same response, trauma also confuses and sometimes secondary infection. If in doubt, revaccinate; with no reaction, always revaccinate.

B. Control of the infected individual, contacts and environment:

1. Report to local health authority: Case report universally required by international regulation, Class 1 (p. 6).
2. Isolation: Hospital isolation in screened wards or rooms until all scabs and crusts have disappeared.
3. Concurrent disinfection: Oral and nasal discharges to be deposited in a paper bag or other suitable container and burned. All articles associated with the patient to be sterilized by high pressure steam or by boiling.
4. Terminal disinfection: Thorough cleaning of sick room and furniture; sterilization of mattress, pillow and bedding.
5. Quarantine: All persons living or working on the same premises as the person who develops smallpox, or otherwise having intensive exposure, should be considered contacts, and promptly vaccinated or revaccinated, or quarantined for 16 days from last exposure. If such contacts are considered immune by reason of prior attack or successful revaccination within the previous 3 years, they should be kept under surveillance until the height of the reaction to the recent vaccination has passed. If the contact is not considered immune, he should be kept under surveillance until 16 days have passed since last contact. Any rise of temperature during surveillance calls for prompt isolation until smallpox can be excluded.
6. Immunization: Prompt vaccination of all contacts, casual as well as intimate, with a potent vaccine.
7. Investigation of contacts and source of infection: The immediately prior case should be sought assiduously. Adults with chickenpox or patients with hemorrhagic or pustular lesions of the skin, particularly those associated in time or place with known smallpox, need careful review for errors in diagnosis.
8. Specific treatment: None.

C. Epidemic measures:

1. Hospital care of patients and suspects until no longer communicable.
2. Careful listing of all contacts and rigorous enforcement of quarantine until protected by successful vaccination; surveillance for 16 days from last exposure.
3. Immediate publicity by all available methods, giving a simple, clear and frank statement of the situation and urging all individuals in the area to be vaccinated. Provide potent vaccine to physicians and hospitals; establish vaccination clinics for those without a private physician.

4. Mass immunization of whole populations of a community or larger area is an emergency measure to be used when smallpox has entered a community and given evidence of material spread.

D. International measures:

1. Telegraphic notification of WHO and adjacent countries by governments of the existence of an epidemic of smallpox.

2. Measures applicable to ships, aircraft and land transport arriving from smallpox areas are specified in International Sanitary Regulations (WHO Techn. Rept. Ser. No. 41, Geneva, 1951).

3. International travellers: Evidence of a previous attack of smallpox or of recent vaccination is a widely enforced requirement for entrance to or departure from a country. The validity of an international certificate of vaccination against smallpox extends for a period of 3 years beginning 8 days after the date of a successful primary vaccination, or in the event of a revaccination, on the date of that revaccination.

SPOROTRICHOSIS

1 *Identification.*—In commonest form, a localized fungus infection of the skin, beginning as a nodule which ultimately forms a black necrotic ulcer. As the nodule grows, lymphatics draining the area gradually become firm and cordlike, with a series of nodules which in turn may soften and ulcerate. Other forms of sporotrichosis occur, such as skeletal, visceral, and disseminated, but are rare in the United States. A fatal result is uncommon.

Laboratory confirmation is through cultivation of the fungus, rarely through observation in direct smear.

2. *Etiologic agent.*—Sporotrichum schenckii, a fungus.

3. *Source and reservoir of infection.*—Presumable source is plants, most likely those with thorns or barbs; reservoir, presumably plants. Infection is common in domestic animals.

4. *Mode of transmission.*—Introduction of fungus through skin following pricks by thorns or barbs, by slivers from wood or lumber, or through skin lesions of persons handling contaminated dressings of patients.

5. *Incubation period.*—The lymphatic form may develop three weeks to three months after injury.

6. *Period of communicability.*—Unknown.

7. *Susceptibility and resistance.*—Man probably is highly susceptible.

8. *Occurrence.*—Cases have been reported from all parts of the world, males more frequently than females, and incidence in adults is higher than in children; reportedly an occupational disease of horticulturists. No differences in racial susceptibility. The disease is characteristically sporadic, and relatively uncommon.

9. *Methods of control:*

A. Preventive measures: Treatment of lumber with fungicides in industries where disease occurs.

B. Control of the infected individual, contacts and environment:
1. Report to local health authority: Official report ordinarily not justifiable, Class 5 (p. 7).
2. Isolation: None.
3. Concurrent disinfection: Of discharges and dressings.
4. Terminal disinfection: Thorough cleaning.
5. Quarantine: None.
6. Immunization: None.
7. Investigation of contacts and source of infection: Not profitable.
8. Specific treatment: Iodides are effective.

C. Epidemic measures: The only reported epidemic involved some 3,000 persons among gold mine workers of South Africa. Control measures included spraying of timbers used in the mine with a mixture of zinc sulphate and triolith.

D. International measures: None.

STREPTOCOCCAL INFECTIONS, HEMOLYTIC

Group A hemolytic streptococci cause a wide variety of conditions differentiated clinically according to portal of entry and tissue of localization of the infectious agent, and presence or absence of a scarlatinal rash. The more important conditions are:

A. Scarlet Fever and Streptococcal Sore Throat (Streptococcal Tonsillitis, Streptococcal Nasopharyngitis).
B. Erysipelas.
C. Puerperal infection.

Streptococcal infections, other than those just mentioned but caused by the same strains of Group A streptococci, include: cellulitis, lymphadenitis, mastoiditis, osteomyelitis, otitis media, peritonitis, septicemia, and various skin and wound infections. Those characterized by purulent exudates are most likely to spread infection, but others such as septicemia are also important because of frequent association with upper respiratory streptococcal carrier states. Insofar as these clinical categories are caused by Group A streptococci, they are different manifestations of the same infectious agent, and therefore should be treated together in their epidemiologic relationships. They constitute an epidemiologic entity, and similar principles of control hold generally for the group.

A. Scarlet Fever and Streptococcal Sore Throat (Streptococcal Tonsillitis, Streptococcal Nasopharyngitis)

1. *Identification.*—Scarlet fever is ordinarily streptococcal sore throat in which the infectious agent is capable of producing erythrogenic toxin and the patient has relatively no antitoxic immunity. If the organism is not a good toxin producer, or if the patient is immune to the toxin, the rash does not occur and streptococcal sore throat results. The distinguishing characteristics are fever, sore throat, exudative

tonsillitis or pharyngitis, tender cervical adenopathy, leucocytosis, enanthem, strawberry tongue and rash (exanthem). Infection and edema of the pharynx involve the faucial pillars and soft palate, often extending to the hard palate; petechiae are sometimes seen against the background of diffuse redness. Tonsils, if present, often show the exudate of acute follicular tonsillitis. The rash is usually a fine erythema, commonly punctate, blanching on pressure and appearing most often on the neck, chest, in the folds of the axilla, elbow and groin and on the inner aspects of the thighs. Typically the rash does not involve the face except in Negroes, but there is flushing of cheeks and circumoral pallor. High fever, nausea, and vomiting accompany severe infections. The desquamation of convalescence is seen at the tips of the fingers and toes and less often over wide areas of the trunk and limbs, including palms and soles. Scarlet fever and streptococcal sore throat may be accompanied or followed by suppurative complications such as otitis media and peritonsillar abscess, and may be followed at an interval of 1 to 4 weeks by non-suppurative complications such as rheumatic fever and glomerulonephritis. Scarlet fever occasionally occurs in patients with other types of streptococcal infections, such as infected wounds. Severity of the disease has been decreasing in the United States for unknown reasons, fatality is low, about one death for each 300 to 400 reported cases. Fatality rates in some parts of the world are 3 to 5%.

Streptococcal sore throat is scarlet fever infection without a rash. The manifestations of this clinical entity are similar to scarlet fever, except that toxic manifestations including rash do not occur, nor does desquamation follow.

Laboratory diagnostic aids include demonstration of a typable Group A streptococcus as the predominant organism in cultures of the throat, and a rise in serum antibody titer (antistreptolysin O, antistreptokinase) from acute to convalescent phase of the illness.

2. *Etiologic agent.*—Streptococcus pyogenes, Group A streptococci, of at least 40 serologically distinct types which vary greatly in geographic and time distributions. Two immunologically different types (A and B) of erythrogenic toxin have been demonstrated.

3. *Source and reservoir of infection.*—Discharges from nose, throat or purulent complications of acutely ill or convalescent patients or carriers, or objects contaminated with such discharges. Nasal carriers are particularly liable to contaminate their environment.

4. *Mode of transmission.*—Transmission is by direct contact with patient or carrier, or by indirect contact through objects handled, or by droplet spread whereby streptococci are inhaled; casual contact rarely leads to infection. Streptococci reach the air via contaminated floor dust, lint from bedclothing, personal clothing, handkerchiefs, or occasionally in droplet nuclei discharged by coughing or sneezing; the importance of air-borne transmission and contamination of the environment in spread of infection has not been clearly established. Explosive outbreaks may follow the ingestion of contaminated milk or other food.

5. *Incubation period.*—Short, usually 2 to 5 days.

6. *Period of communicability.*—In uncomplicated cases, during incubation and clinical illness, approximately 10 days. Thereafter in untreated patients, communicability decreases progressively, becoming negli-

gible in 2 to 3 weeks although a carrier state may persist for months. Persons with untreated complications resulting in purulent discharges may spread infection for weeks or months. Adequate treatment with penicillin will eliminate probability of transmission from patients or carriers within 24 hours.

7. *Susceptibility and resistance.*—Susceptibility is general, although many persons develop either antitoxic or type-specific antibacterial immunity, or both, through inapparent infection. Antibacterial immunity develops only against the type of Group A streptococcus which induces the patient's disease or inapparent infection, and lasts at least several years. Second attacks of streptococcal sore throat, due to a different type of streptococcus, are not uncommon. The frequency of inapparent infection is unknown, but undoubtedly is related to the prevalence of streptococci, and possibly to the type of streptococcus.

Immunity against erythrogenic toxin, and hence to rash, develops within a week of the onset of scarlet fever and is usually permanent. Second attacks of scarlet fever are rare but may occur because of the two immunological forms of toxin.

Both active and passive immunization against erythrogenic toxin are possible but not practical. Neither active nor passive immunization against the streptococcus itself can be accomplished satisfactorily at the present time.

8. *Occurrence.*—Clinical disease is most common in temperate zones, less common in semi-tropical areas and rare in tropical climates. Inapparent infections are as common or more common in the tropics than in temperate zones.

In the United States, epidemiological behavior may be endemic, epidemic, or sporadic. Epidemic occurrence is more frequent in certain geographic areas, such as New England, the Great Lakes region and the Rocky Mountain area. Apart from food-borne epidemics, which may occur in any season, the highest incidence is during late winter and spring; generally in the 5–9 year age group; no sex or racial susceptibilities have been defined. Scarlet fever has followed a similar pattern in central Europe, the Scandinavian countries and Spain during the past two decades.

9. *Methods of control:*

A. Preventive measures:

1. Provision for throat cultures, with isolation of hemolytic streptococci and identification of serologic group and type.
2. Emphasis on the fact that absence of rash does not decrease the danger of streptococcal infection.
3. Boiling or pasteurization of milk.
4. Exclusion of infected persons from handling milk or other food likely to be contaminated.
5. Milk from any cow with evidence of mastitis should be excluded from sale or use.
6. Chemoprophylaxis with oral sulfonamide drugs (0.5 to 1.0 gram per day) or penicillin (200,000 to 250,000 units twice a day on an empty stomach) for persons in whom recurrent streptococcal infection provides a special risk, such as individuals who have had rheumatic fever or chorea within 5 years or are under 18 years of age. See Rheumatic Fever (p. 148). When streptococcal disease

occurs in a household which includes a patient with rheumatic fever or person with history of that disease, all members of the family should receive a therapeutic course of penicillin.

B. Control of the infected individual, contacts, and environment:

Control of streptococcal infections depends on preventing the dissemination of Group A streptococci and their implantation in the tissues of susceptible subjects.

1. Report to local health authority: Case report of scarlet fever required in most states and countries, Class 2A (p. 7). Notification of streptococcal sore throat is inaccurate and of limited value in control because of difficulty in diagnosis and differentiation from non-bacterial exudative tonsillitis and pharyngitis; recommended that reporting be limited to epidemics, Class 4 (p. 7).

2. Isolation: In order of preference, in a single room, cubicle or small ward; in uncomplicated cases until clinical recovery or not less than 7 days from onset. Isolation may be terminated after 24 hours treatment with penicillin, provided therapy is continued for 7 to 10 days.

3. Concurrent disinfection: Of purulent discharges and all articles soiled therewith.

4. Terminal disinfection: Thorough cleaning; sunning or other treatment of blankets.

5. Quarantine: None.

6. Immunization: None.

7. Investigation of contacts and source of infection: Not indicated in sporadic cases.

8. Specific treatment: Penicillin; various forms (aqueous penicillin, dibenzyl esters of penicillin) are all effective when administered parenterally. Penicillin G by mouth may be effective. Therapy should be started early and continued for 10 days. Such treatment will ameliorate the acute illness, reduce the frequency of suppurative complications, and prevent the development of rheumatic fever and acute glomerulonephritis. The tetracycline antibiotics may be employed for patients sensitive to penicillin, but therapy must be continued for 10 days. Sulfonamide drugs are not recommended; scarlet fever antitoxin and pooled convalescent human serum are rarely used.

C. Epidemic measures:

1. Determine source and manner of spread, as person-to-person, by milk, or food-borne. Outbreaks can often be traced to an individual or animal with a persistent streptoccal infection through identification of the serologic type of streptococcus.

2. With limited population groups or under special circumstances, penicillin prophylaxis may be given to intimate and household contacts, to those known to have been exposed to contaminated milk or other food, or to the entire population group (see 9A6). In the latter circumstance, sulfonamide drugs should not be administered for prolonged periods because of likelihood that resistant strains of streptococci will develop.

3. Prompt investigation of any group of cases as to possibility of contaminated milk with exclusion of suspected milk supply from sale or use until pasteurized. Contamination of milk or food can occasionally or under special circumstances be determined by culture.

D. International measures : None.

B. Erysipelas

1. *Identification.*—An acute infection characterized by fever, constitutional symptoms, leucocytosis, and a red, tender edematous, spreading lesion of the skin, often with a definite raised border. The central point of origin tends to clear as the periphery extends. Face and legs are common sites. Recurrences are frequent. The disease may be especially severe, with bacteremia, in patients suffering from debilitating disease. Fatality varies greatly with part of body affected and according to associated disease. Rates of 1 to 2% are now common in hospital practice.

Group A streptococci may be isolated from the margin of the skin lesion, the nose and throat, and occasionally from the blood.

Erysipelas due to Group A streptococci is to be distinguished from erysipeloid, caused by Erysipelothrix rhusiopathiae, a localized cutaneous infection, primarily an occupational disease of persons handling animals, meat, fish, poultry and shellfish.

2. *Etiologic agent.*—Streptococcus pyogenes, Group A streptococci, of at least 40 types. No specific strain or type has been shown to cause erysipelas.

3. *Source and reservoir of infection.*—Persons infected with Group A streptococci, with the source either respiratory discharges of the same individual or of exogenous origin.

4. *Mode of transmission.*—Transmission is by direct contact with patient or carrier, by indirect contact through objects handled, or by droplet spread whereby streptococci are inhaled. Streptococci reach the air through contaminated floor dust, lint from bedclothing, personal clothing, handkerchiefs, or occasionally in droplet nuclei discharged by coughing or sneezing. The importance of air-borne transmission has not been established. Erysipelas may be associated epidemiologically with other forms of Group A streptococcal infection.

5. *Incubation period.*—Unknown ; probably not more than 2 days.

6. *Period of communicability.*—Unknown ; presumably until clinical recovery, about 10 days in untreated patients. Adequate treatment with penicillin will eliminate probability of transmission from patients or carriers within 24 hours.

7. *Susceptibility and resistance.*—Susceptibility is greatest in infants, in older persons and in the debilitated. One attack appears to predispose to subsequent attacks ; recurrences may be due to streptococcal infection or to hypersensitivity. Whether or not type-specific immunity occurs is unknown. No available immunization procedures.

8. *Occurrence.*—Geographic and seasonal distributions are similar to scarlet fever and streptococcal sore throat. Common after 20 years of age with highest attack rates at 40 to 60 years, and frequently in infants. No clear predilection for sex or race has been defined. Occurrence is sporadic, even during epidemics of streptococcal infection.

9. *Methods of control:*

   A. Preventive measures:

      1. Personal cleanliness and avoidance of transferring the infectious agent to the broken skin.

      2. Chemoprophylaxis with oral sulfonamide drugs or penicillin as for scarlet fever and streptococcal sore throat.

      3. Recurrence of erysipelas may be prevented by administration of oral sulfonamide drugs or penicillin during and after convalescence, but may need to be continued for months or years depending on the individual situation.

   B. Control of the infected individual, contacts and environment:

      1. Report to local health authority: Obligatory report of epidemics; no individual case report, Class 4 (p. 7).

      2. Isolation: During period of communicability; patients are a potential danger to young infants and to surgical and obstetrical patients. Isolation may be terminated after 24 hours treatment with penicillin, provided therapy is continued for 7 to 10 days.

      3. Concurrent disinfection: Of dressings and discharges from lesions.

      4. Terminal disinfection: Thorough cleaning; sunning or other treatment of blankets.

      5. Quarantine: None.

      6. Immunization: None.

      7. Investigation of contacts and source of infection: None.

      8. Specific treatment: Penicillin; procaine penicillin is preferred but oral penicillin G has been used; continue for 7 to 10 days. The tetracycline antibiotics or sulfonamide drugs may be substituted if patient is sensitive to penicillin.

   C. Epidemic measures: Erysipelas is now rarely epidemic in the western world. In the event of an outbreak in a limited population group, institution or hospital, prophylactic administration of penicillin or sulfonamide drugs, as outlined under scarlet fever and streptococcal sore throat.

   D. International measures: None.

C. Streptococcal Puerperal Fever (Puerperal Septicemia)

1. *Identification.*—An acute infection, usually febrile, accompanied by local and general symptoms and signs of bacterial invasion of the genital tract and sometimes of the blood of the postpartum or postabortum patient. Fatality for streptococcal puerperal fever is negligible when adequately treated.

   The causative agent can be recovered by bacterial culture of vaginal discharges, cervix and blood and identified by bacteriologic and serologic methods.

   A goodly proportion of puerperal infections are of other origin than hemolytic streptococci. They are to be differentiated by appropriate bacteriological means, for they are clinically similar. The infecting microorganisms include a variety of bacterial agents, non-hemolytic streptococci, anaerobic streptococci, Staphylococcus aureus, Escherichia coli, Clostridium welchii, Bacteroides sp., and others. Group A streptococci are of primary importance in postpartum infection; the anaerobic organisms, colon bacilli and staphylococci in postabortum infections. Treatment of infections caused by bacteria other than hemolytic streptococci is by appropriate antibiotics; the fatality is somewhat greater. Epidemiologic characteristics and methods of control now described for Group A streptococcal infections apply equally to the others.

2. *Etiologic agent.*—Streptococcus pyogenes, Group A hemolytic streptococci; hemolytic streptococci of Groups B, C, D, and G. Mixed infections with other bacteria are common.

3. *Source and reservoir of infection.*—From an external source or from the respiratory tract, intestinal tract, genital tract, or skin of the patient. In postpartum infections due to Group A streptococci, the organism comes from an attendant in about half of cases, from a familial contact in about one-fifth, and from the patient's respiratory tract in the remainder. In postabortum infections, the organism most frequently comes from the patient herself due to faulty or inadequate aseptic technic.

4. *Mode of transmission.*—Direct transfer of infectious agent to uterus may be accomplished by hands or by instruments used in examinations before, during or following parturition or abortion; transfer of organisms to the genital tract from nose and throat of a carrier or infected attendant, or from the patient's respiratory tract, intestinal tract or skin, is usually by the hands; indirectly as for other streptococcal and wound infections.

5. *Incubation period.*—One to three days, rarely longer.

6. *Period of communicability.*—During persistence of infectious discharges from genital tract of the patient. Infectiousness of the patient herself, in the case of Group A streptococcal infection, will become negligible after 24 to 48 hours of adequate penicillin therapy. In institutional outbreaks contamination of the environment may be extensive and persistent for days or weeks.

7. *Susceptibility and resistance.*—Susceptibility is general. The birth process and the abortion procedure increase the opportunity for implantation of pathogenic bacteria.

8. *Occurrence.*—Worldwide in distribution but reliable morbidity data are not available. In the United States, mortality has declined more than 80% in the past 15 years, and the fatality has dropped precipitously since the advent of antibiotic drugs; greater for white than non-white races. Similar changes have occurred throughout the western world. Now is chiefly a sporadic disease, although epidemics may occur in institutions where aseptic technics are faulty.

9. *Methods of control:*

   A. Preventive measures:

   1. Maintenance of high standards of prenatal care and extension of such services to all segments of the population.
   2. Strict asepsis in obstetrical procedures with special attention to possible contamination from mouth and nose of attendants as well as by hands and instruments.
   3. Protection of patient during labor and postpartum from attendants, visitors and other patients with respiratory or skin infection.
   4. Bacteriologic search for carriers among attendants, physicians, nurses, and nursemaids.

5. Prophylactic use of antibiotic drugs in patients undergoing difficult deliveries or sustaining complications that predispose to infection, such as premature rupture of membranes, severe lacerations or retained products of conception.

6. Education of women in the hazards of self-interruption of pregnancy.

B. Control of the infected individual, contacts and environment:

1. Report to local health authority: Obligatory report of epidemics; no individual case report, Class 4 (p. 7).

2. Isolation: Strict isolation while infectious discharges persist. In patients with Group A streptococcal infection, isolation may be terminated after 24 hours treatment with penicillin, provided therapy is continued for 7 to 10 days.

3. Concurrent disinfection: Of dressings and discharges.

4. Terminal disinfection: Thorough cleaning; sunning or other treatment of blankets.

5. Quarantine: None.

6. Immunization: None.

7. Investigation of contacts and source of infection: Serologic typing of strains of Group A streptococci is of value in tracing the source of infection.

8. Specific treatment: Penicillin as for other streptococcal infections (see Scarlet Fever 9B8, p. 171). Strict aseptic technic must be used in examination, obtaining of cultures or surgical interference since all vaginal manipulations increase the danger of reinfection or of introduction of new organisms.

C. Epidemic measures: The most probable cause of an epidemic of puerperal infection is a Group A streptococcus and the most likely location is a hospital or maternity home. General asepsis should be strictly enforced. The identity and source of the infecting strain of streptococcus should be determined. Infected attendants or carriers should be treated with penicillin. Other personnel and patients may be given oral penicillin prophylactically (200,000 to 250,000 units twice a day on an empty stomach and continued until the epidemic has subsided).

D. International measures: None.

STRONGYLOIDIASIS

1. *Identification.*—An infection with the nematode Strongyloides stercoralis usually located in the mucosa of the duodenum and upper jejunum. Clinical manifestations include dermatitis when the larvae are penetrating the skin, usually of the feet; cough and rales, or even pneumonitis when they are passing through the lungs; abdominal symptoms when the adult females are in the mucosa of the intestine. Symptoms may be mild or severe, depending upon the intensity of the infection. Abdominal symptoms in order of frequency are pain, usually epigastric and often suggesting peptic ulcer, nausea, weight

loss, vomiting, diarrhea, weakness, and constipation. Urticaria may occur, especially with reinfection. In rare cases internal auto-infection with hyperparasitism may lead to wasting and death. Eosinophilia is usually moderate, may be absent or intense.

Diagnosis is by identifying motile larvae in freshly passed feces, or eggs and motile larvae in fluids obtained by duodenal intubation. Held at room temperature for 24 hours or longer, feces may show developing stages of the parasite, including filariform or infective larvae and non-parasitic male and female adults.

2. *Etiologic agent.*—Strongyloides stercoralis.

3. *Source and reservoir of infection.*—Infective (filariform) larvae in moist soil contaminated with feces deposited by infected person or dog.

4. *Mode of transmission.*—Infective or filariform larvae penetrate the skin, usually of the foot, and are carried to the lungs, where further development takes place. They penetrate the capillary walls, enter the alveoli, ascend the trachea to the epiglottis and descend the digestive tract to the upper part of the small intestine where development of the adult female is completed, these females being generally held to be parthenogenetic. They live embedded in the mucosa of the intestine where eggs are deposited and promptly hatch, liberating rhabditiform larvae which migrate into the lumen of the intestine, leave the host with feces, and develop either into infective filariform larvae or free-living adults. Fertilized females produce eggs which soon hatch, liberating rhabditiform larvae, which become filariform larvae.

5. *Incubation period.*—From penetration of skin by filariform larvae until rhabditiform larvae appear in feces is about 17 days.

6. *Period of communicability.*—As long as living worms remain in the intestine.

7. *Susceptibility and resistance.*—Susceptibility to infection is universal. Acquired immunity to strongyloidiasis has been demonstrated in laboratory animals but not in man.

8. *Occurrence.*—Geographic distribution closely parallels that of hook-worm disease, but apparently indigenous cases occur far beyond the confines of ancylostomiasis, e.g. Boston, Massachusetts, and Winnipeg, Manitoba. Prevalence in any endemic area is not accurately known.

9. *Methods of control:*

    A. Preventive measures:

        1. As for Ancylostomiasis (p. 22). The installation and strict use of sanitary disposal systems for human excreta, particularly sanitary privies in rural areas, are fundamental preventive measures.

        2. Rigid attention to hygienic habits, particularly the wearing of shoes.

    B. Control of the infected individual, contacts and environment:

        1. Report to local health authority: In selected endemic areas; in most states and countries not a reportable disease, Class 3C (p. 7).

        2. Isolation: None.

        3. Concurrent disinfection: Sanitary disposal of excreta.

        4. Terminal disinfection: None.

5. Quarantine: None.
6. Immunization: None.
7. Investigation of contacts and source of infection: Of family contacts for evidence of infection.
8. Specific treatment: Gentian violet medicinal is usually employed, but rarely eliminates the infection.

C. Epidemic measures: Not applicable, a sporadic infection.

D. International measures: None.

SYPHILIS

Two distinctive forms of syphilis are recognized. That form which is venereally spread is of worldwide occurrence. The other, often referred to as endemic syphilis or bejel, is of non-venereal spread and confined to parts of the world where economic, social and climatic conditions favor its development; not seen in the United States.

A. Venereal Syphilis

1. *Identification.*—An acute and chronic relapsing treponematosis characterized clinically by a primary lesion, a secondary eruption involving skin and mucous membranes, long periods of latency, and late lesions of skin, bone, viscera, the central nervous and cardiovascular systems. The primary lesion appears at about 3 weeks as a papule, and after erosion presents a variety of forms, the most distinctive although not the most frequent being an indurated chancre; invasion of the blood precedes the initial lesion; a hard non-fluctuant painless satellite bubo commonly follows. Infection without chancre is fairly frequent. During the next 4 to 6 weeks, even without specific treatment the chancre begins to involute and the generalized secondary eruption appears, often accompanied by mild constitutional symptoms. Secondary manifestations disappear spontaneously within a few weeks to as long as 12 months, with subsequent clinical latency of weeks to years, often interrupted in early years by recurrence of infectious lesions of skin and mucous membrane or developing lesions of the eye and central nervous system; in later years (5 to 20) by explosive destructive non-infectious lesions of skin, bone and mucosal surfaces. Latency sometimes continues through life, sometimes spontaneous recovery occurs and in other instances and unpredictably late disabling manifestations of cardiovascular, central nervous or other system appear. The actual fatality is unknown; prenatal infection is frequently fatal, before birth or in infancy. Early acquired syphilis does not result in death or serious disability but the late manifestations shorten life, impair health and limit occupational efficiency.

Primary and secondary syphilis are confirmed by dark-field examination of exudates of lesions; in all instances by serologic tests for syphilis through examination of blood and spinal fluid. These tests may be supplemented by treponemal immobilization or agglutination tests to aid in the exclusion of biologic false positive reactions.

2. *Etiologic agent.*—Treponema pallidum.

3. *Source and reservoir of infection.*—Exudates from obvious or concealed moist early lesions of skin and mucous membrane of infected per-

sons; body fluids and secretions (saliva, semen, blood, vaginal discharges) during infectious period.

4. *Mode of transmission.*—By direct contact (sexual intercourse, kissing, fondling of children) during primary and secondary syphilis. Transmission through indirect contact with contaminated articles has relatively little significance. Prenatal infection may occur after but not before the fourth month of pregnancy through placental transfer of treponemata.

5. *Incubation period.*—Ten days to 10 weeks, usually 3 weeks.

6. *Period of communicability.*—Variable and not definitely known; during primary and secondary stages and during mucocutaneous recurrence which may occur intermittently during 2 to 4 years. Extent of communicability through sexual intercourse during early latent period (2 to 4 years) has not been established; the possibility of inapparent lesions requires that this stage be considered potentially infectious.

7. *Susceptibility and resistance.*—Susceptibility is universal; no natural immunity. Infection leads to gradually developing resistance against the homologous strain and to an extent against heterologous strains of treponema; may be overcome by large reinfecting doses or fail to develop by reason of early treatment. Superinfection may produce lesions simulating those of the currently existing stage; in late latency, superinfection has special significance through ability to produce benign late lesions of skin and mucous membrane.

8. *Occurrence.*—One of the more frequent communicable diseases; widespread throughout the world and primarily involving young persons between ages 15 and 30 years. The considerable differences in racial incidence are related more to social than to biologic factors.

9. *Methods of control:*

A. Preventive measures. The following are applicable to all venereal diseases: syphilis, chancroid, lymphogranuloma venereum, granuloma inguinale and gonorrhea.

1. General health promotional measures, health and sex education, preparation for marriage, premarital and prenatal examinations as part of general physical examination. Improvement of social and economic conditions, including recreational facilities.

2. Protection of the community by suppression of commercialized prostitution and of clandestine sexual promiscuity, in cooperation with social and law enforcement agencies; by teaching methods of personal prophylaxis applicable before, during and after exposure; by repeated prenatal serologic examination of all pregnant women.

3. Provision of facilities for early diagnosis and treatment; encouragement of their use through education of the public concerning symptoms of the venereal diseases and modes of spread, and through making these services available irrespective of economic status of the infected person. Intensive case-finding programs, to include interview of patients and tracing of contacts, and repeated mass serologic examination of special groups with known high incidence of venereal disease.

4. An emphasis on control of patients with venereal disease in a transmissible stage should not preclude search for per-

sons past that stage; has value in preventing relapse, congenital syphilis and disability due to late manifestations.

B. Control of the infected individual, contacts and environment:

1. Report to local health authority: Case report is required in all states of the United States and variously in other countries, Class 2B (p. 7). Reporting in the United States is commonly too incomplete to be a reliable guide to administrative practice. Accurate reporting has increasing value as syphilis declines, as a means to determine the amount of effort to be expended on control activities.

2. Isolation: None; modern therapy limits communicability to 24 hours or less. To avoid reinfection, patients should refrain from sexual intercourse with previous partners not under treatment.

3. Concurrent disinfection: None in adequately treated cases; care in disposal of discharges from open lesions and articles soiled therewith.

4. Terminal disinfection: None.

5. Quarantine: None.

6. Immunization: None.

7. Investigation of contacts and source of infection: Interview of patients and tracing of contacts are the fundamental features of a program for control of venereal disease. Trained interviewers obtain the best results. The stage of the disease determines criteria for contact tracing: (a) for primary syphilis, all sex contacts of preceding 3 months; (b) for secondary syphilis, those of the preceding 6 months; (c) for early latent syphilis, those of the preceding 1 year provided time of primary and secondary lesions is not established; (d) for late and late latent syphilis, marital partners and children of infected mothers; (e) for congenital syphilis, all members of immediate family.

8. Specific treatment: Penicillin; dosage depends on stage of disease and whether on an individual or mass control basis. In general, large amounts should be given initially on the day of diagnosis to assure reasonably effective therapy if the patient fails to return. Consideration should be given to a plan whereby a full course of antibiotic therapy is given immediately to sexual contacts of patients with proved primary or secondary syphilis in order to abort or cure possible disease.

C. Epidemic measures: Intensification of measures outlined under 9A and 9B.

D. International measures:

1. Appropriate examination of groups of adolescents and young adults moving from areas of high prevalence of treponemal infections.

2. Adherence to agreements among nations (e.g. Brussels agreement) as to records, and provision of diagnostic, treatment and contact interviewing facilities at seaports for foreign seamen engaged in maritime commerce.

3. Provision for rapid international exchange of information on contacts.

B. Non-Venereal Syphilis

1. *Identification.*—Endemic syphilis and bejel are diseases of limited geographical distribution, acute nature, predominantly household occurrence, and characterized clinically by an eruption of skin and mucous membrane, usually without evident initial primary sore. Early skin lesions, indistinguishable from those of venereal syphilis, are macular or papular, often hypertrophic and frequently circinate; mucous patches of the mouth often appear first, soon followed by moist papules in folds of skin and by drier lesions on trunk and extremities. Plantar and palmar hyperkeratoses frequently occur in bejel, often with painful fissuring; a patchy depigmentation and hyperpigmentation of the skin, and alopecia, are common. Inflammatory or destructive lesions of skin, long bones and nasopharynx are late manifestations. Unlike venereal syphilis, the nervous and cardiovascular systems seem rarely to be involved. The fatality is negligible. Synonyms: Sibbens, Radesyke.

   Serologic tests for syphilis are reactive in the early stages and remain so for many years of latency, gradually tending toward non-reactivity; response to treatment as in venereal syphilis.

2. *Etiologic agent.*—Treponema pallidum.

3. *Source and reservoir of infection.*—Infected persons; surfaces and exudates of early lesions of skin and mucous membrane.

4. *Mode of transmission.*—Direct household or other contact with infectious lesions, as favored by common eating and drinking utensils and household crowding under substandard hygienic conditions. Flies, lice and fleas are possible factors. Congenital transmission is rare.

5. *Incubation period.*—2 weeks to 3 months, usually about 6 weeks.

6. *Period of communicability.*—During the period of moist eruptions of skin and until mucous patches disappear; may extend over several weeks or months.

7. *Susceptibility and resistance.*—Similar to venereal syphilis.

8. *Occurrence.*—A common disease in localized areas; known as endemic syphilis in the Balkans and in Turkey, and as bejel in Eastern Mediterranean regions. These two conditions resemble each other in practically all respects, occurring equally in the two sexes and primarily among infants and young children. An apparently similar syndrome has been reported by other names in various parts of the world.

9. *Methods of control.*—The considerable decline in overt early venereal syphilis throughout much of the world calls for particular attention to non-venereal treponematoses, not yet under control, and including Yaws, p. 208 and Pinta, p. 125.

   A. Preventive measures:

       1. Those of the non-venereal treponematoses. See Yaws 9A, p. 208.

   B. Control of the infected individual, contacts and environment:

       1. Report to local health authority: In selected endemic areas; in most countries not a reportable disease, Class 3B (p. 7).

    2. See Yaws 9B for Items 2–8, applicable to all non-venereal treponematoses.

C. Epidemic measures: Intensification of preventive and control activities.

D. International measures: See Yaws 9D.

TAENIASIS AND CYSTICERCOSIS

1. *Identification.*—Taenias infection of man is manifest in two forms, the one a benign intestinal infection with the adult worm of two species, beef and pork tapeworms, and the other a severe somatic disease (cysticercosis) of many different tissues arising through localization of larvae of the pork tapeworm.

    Clinical manifestations of infection with the adult worm are variable, frequently vague or absent, sometimes nervousness, insomnia, anorexia, loss of weight, abdominal pain, and digestive disturbances. A non-fatal disease. Synonym: Beef or Pork Tapeworm Infection.

    Infection with adult tapeworms is confirmed through identification of proglottides (segments) of the worm or of eggs in feces. Specific diagnosis is through morphological characters of the gravid proglottides (Strobila), usually obtained after treatment; obtaining the scolex or head confirms the identification and assures elimination of the worm.

    If eggs of the pork tapeworm are swallowed by man, they will hatch in the small intestine and the larval forms (cysticerci) will develop in the subcutaneous tissues, striated muscles and other regions of the body. Grave consequences can ensue when they localize in heart, eye or central nervous system. Recognition of subcutaneous or somatic cysticercosis is by excision of the larva and microscopic examination. In the presence of cerebral symptoms, somatic cysticercosis strongly suggests cerebral involvement. Roentgen ray examination is helpful in locating calcified cysticerci in the brain and somatic muscles, and in determining the intensity of infection. A chronic disease with ultimate high fatality.

    Other species, including Hymenolepis nana, the common dwarf tapeworm, and H. diminuta, and Dipylidium caninum, are relatively rare adult tapeworms of man, have doubtful pathogenicity, but the eggs must be differentiated from taenia eggs.

2. *Etiologic agent.*—Taenia saginata, the beef tapeworm of man, intestinal infection with adult worm only; Taenia solium, the pork tapeworm of man, intestinal infection with adult worm and somatic infection with larvae (cysticercosis).

3. *Source and reservoir of infection.*—Immediate source of infection for Taenia saginata is the flesh of infected cattle; reservoir is feces of an infected person. For intestinal taeniasis due to Taenia solium the source of infection is the flesh of infected pigs, and the reservoir is feces of infected persons.

4. *Mode of transmission.*—For Taenia saginata, by ingestion of raw or inadequately cooked beef containing the infective larva—a cysticercus. For Taenia solium (1) by ingestion of raw or inadequately cooked

pork containing the infective larva (cysticercus) resulting in the development of the adult worm in the intestine; or (2) by direct hand to mouth transfer of eggs in feces, or indirectly through ingestion of food or water contaminated with eggs, resulting in somatic cysticercosis.

5. *Incubation period.*—Eight to ten weeks.

6. *Period of communicability.*—The adult worm of Taenia saginata is not transmissible from man to man; eggs are disseminated in the environment as long as man harbors the worm in the intestine. Man disseminates eggs of Taenia solium as long as the worm is harbored in the intestine. Transmission of adult worms from man to man is impossible.

7. *Susceptibility and resistance.*—Man is universally susceptible. No apparent resistance follows infection.

8. *Occurrence.*—Cosmopolitan distribution; particularly prevalent wherever beef or pork is eaten raw or slightly cooked. Incidence is highest in tropical countries and in the Slavic countries of Europe. Where Taenia saginata and Taenia solium co-exist, taenia saginata is by far the commoner. Infection with T. solium is rare in the United States and Canada.

9. *Methods of control:*

    A. Preventive measures:

        1. Prevention of soil pollution with human feces in rural areas, improvement in barnyard sanitation, and education of the public.

        2. Thorough cooking of beef and pork insures against infection.

        3. Since cysticercosis in cattle is usually a light infection, meat inspection is of limited value; cysticercosis in swine is often intense and meat inspection can eliminate much infective pork from markets but cannot insure against infection.

        4. Immediate treatment of persons harboring adult Taenia solium is essential to prevent human cysticercosis.

    B. Control of the infected individual, contacts and environment:

        1. Report to local health authority: Official report not ordinarily justifiable, Class 5 (page 7).

        2. Isolation: None. Patients with T. solium infection should be excluded from food preparation and serving.

        3. Concurrent disinfection: Sanitary disposal of feces; for T. solium rigid sanitation with washing of hands after defecating and before eating.

        4. Terminal disinfection: None.

        5. Quarantine: None.

        6. Immunization: None.

        7. Investigation of contacts and source of infection: Usually not a profitable procedure.

        8. Specific treatment: Oleoresin of aspidium is used most commonly for intestinal taeniasis; successful results have been reported with quinacrine. No specific therapy for cysticercosis.

    C. Epidemic measures: None.

    D. International measures: None.

TETANUS

1. *Identification.*—An acute disease induced by toxin of the tetanus bacillus; characterized by painful muscular contractions, primarily of masseter and neck muscles, and secondarily of the trunk; rigidity is sometimes confined to the region of injury. History of injury and known portal of entry sometimes lacking. Much variation in fatality according to age and length of incubation; average about 35%. Tetanus neonatorum is usually through infection of the unhealed umbilicus, with initial general illness of the infant, refusal to nurse, stiffness of the jaws, and later rigid convulsions ending almost invariably in death.

2. *Etiologic agent.*—Clostridium tetani, tetanus bacillus.

3. *Source and reservoir of infection.*—Soil, street dust, and animal feces.

4. *Mode of transmission.*—Direct or indirect inoculation of wound.

5. *Incubation period.*—Commonly 4 days to 3 weeks, dependent somewhat upon the character, extent, and location of the wound; longer periods have been noted. Subsequent operative interference or local tissue changes may initiate activity of quiescent spores at long intervals after the original wound infection.

6. *Period of communicability.*—Not communicable from man to man.

7. *Susceptibility and resistance.*—Susceptibility is general. Active immunity is produced by tetanus toxoid, passive immunity by tetanus antitoxin.

8. *Occurrence.*—World-wide distribution following wound infection, but a relatively uncommon disease. Most frequent in North America among young males and in summer, especially following wounds contaminated with manured soil. The condition is a serious factor in infant mortality where midwives are ignorant or incompetent. A disease of much moment in military practice, now effectively controlled by active immunization.

9. *Methods of control:*

   A. Preventive measures:

      1. Active immunization with tetanus toxoid is desirable for those likely to be exposed to infection with tetanus; advised in infancy or early childhood, preferably combined with appropriate immunizing agents for protection against pertussis, diphtheria or both (see Diphtheria 9A1, p. 51). In addition to the initial inoculation with doses and intervals between injections recommended for the particular form of toxoid used, another (reinforcing) dose should be given 8 to 12 months later, and renewal doses at the time of each injury where danger of tetanus exists. Reinjections in the absence of injury should be at intervals no longer than 5 years. It is also important that the person should have with him at all times a record of his inoculation in case of injury. Tetanus toxoid under such conditions has proved a more effective method of prevention than tetanus antitoxin which is not without danger from sensitivity to horse serum; particularly indicated in persons known to be allergic to a wide range of substances and especially to horse serum. Active immunization of pregnant women with tetanus toxoid is

183

recommended in regions where tetanus neonatorum is prevalent; maternally transmitted passive immunity will protect new born infants.

2. In the absence of previous active immunization with tetanus toxoid, passive protection by tetanus antitoxin is recommended after injury in regions where tetanus is prevalent, and in all instances where contaminated material may be imbedded in a wound; duration about 10 days.

3. Removal from wounds of all foreign matter by thorough cleansing, with debridement where applicable.

4. Extension of preventive methods to persons in industry and on farms.

5. Licensing of midwives authorized to attend confinements, with professional supervision and education as to methods, equipment and the technic of asepsis.

B. Control of the infected individual, contacts and environment:

1. Report to local health authority. Case report required in most states and countries, Class 2A (p. 7).

2. Isolation: None.

3. Quarantine: None.

4. Immunization: In absence of adequate previous inoculation with tetanus toxoid reinforced by another injection of toxoid at the time of injury, a person who has been so wounded that danger of tetanus exists, should receive a subcutaneous injection of tetanus antitoxin, 3,000 units, on the day of the wound. A second injection within 10 days may be desirable in certain instances, but precautions must be taken against developed sensitivity.

5. Investigation of contacts and source of infection: None; the infecting microörganism is widespread.

6. Concurrent disinfection: None.

7. Terminal disinfection: None.

8. Specific treatment: Tetanus antitoxin in a single large dose intravenously; penicillin in large doses intramuscularly. Sedation is the important therapeutic consideration.

C. Epidemic measures: Thorough search for inadequacies in technic of sterilization in the uncommon hospital outbreaks; in tetanus of the newborn, rigid inquiry into competence and licensure of attendants at birth.

D. International measures: Active immunization against tetanus is recommended for international travellers.

TOXOPLASMOSIS

1. *Identification.*—A protozoan infection which may be acquired prenatally from the mother, or at any time of life postnatally. Prenatal infection acquired during gestation may lead to death of the fetus or to manifestations at birth of chorioretinitis, cerebral calcification, hydrocephalus or microcephalus, psychomotor retardation or convulsions. Prenatal infection acquired late in gestation may be manifested after birth by fever, jaundice, rash, hepatomegaly, splenomegaly, xanthrochromic spinal fluid and convulsions. The

chronic manifestations listed above may develop later. Infections acquired after birth may be mild, with no recognized symptoms, or may be manifested by fever, lymphadenopathy and lymphocytosis lasting a few weeks, or may be severe with a generalized exanthem, jaundice, and cerebral manifestations leading rapidly to death.

Definitive diagnosis is by microscopic demonstration of Toxoplasma in body tissues or fluids during life or at autopsy; or in laboratory reared albino mice inoculated with such materials. Laboratory diagnostic aids are complement fixation test and methyleneblue dye test of Sabin and Feldman.

2. *Etiologic agent.*—Toxoplasma gondii.

3. *Source and reservoir of infection.*—The exact source of human infection is not known; the pregnant woman in the primary stage of the infection infects the fetus in utero or possibly during delivery. Rodents, dogs, cats, swine, cattle, sheep, goats and other mammals and birds are reservoirs; a most ubiquitous protozoan parasite.

4. *Mode of transmission.*—Unknown; presumably man becomes infected by ingesting excreta from infected animals or by direct contact with them. Congenital infection is apparently through the placenta. No arthropod vector has been discovered, but certain ticks, infected in the laboratory, have transmitted the infection to experimental animals.

5. *Incubation period.*—Unknown; probably from about 2 weeks to several months.

6. *Period of communicability.*—Probably not communicable from man to man except during period of gestation through the placenta and possibly during delivery. In animals, probably during acute stage or as long as organisms are excreted in feces, urine or saliva.

7. *Susceptibility and Resistance.*—Susceptibility is general. Recovery from one attack probably confers permanent immunity.

8. *Occurrence.*—Worldwide distribution in animals. Serological surveys and recognized clinical cases also indicate worldwide distribution in man. In some areas 50 percent or more of surveyed groups over 20 years of age have positive serological reactions.

9. *Methods of control:*

   A. Preventive measures:

      1. Avoidance of intimate contact with sick animals and birds, avoidance of tick bites, and keeping premises free from rats and mice may prevent infection. No specific preventive measures are known.

   B. Control of the infected individual, contacts and environment:

      1. Report to local health authority: Official report not ordinarily justifiable, Class 5 (p. 7).
      2. Isolation: None.
      3. Concurrent disinfection: None.
      4. Terminal disinfection: None.
      5. Quarantine: None.
      6. Immunization: None.
      7. Investigation of contacts and source of infection: In congenital cases, determine antibodies in mother and other members of family; in acquired cases, determine contact with infected animals and history of tick or insect bite.

8. Specific treatment: In experimental infections of animals, sulfonamides have a prophylactic value, and when administered early have a curative effect. A combination of pyrimethamine (daraprim) with these compounds has given better results. The results in man are little or none.

C. Epidemic measures: Not applicable, a sporadic disease. Community surveys and voluntary reporting by lying-in hospitals for prescribed periods and in particular regions are needed to estimate incidence, and along with thorough case study, to obtain information leading to improved control.

D. International measures: None.

TRACHOMA

1. *Identification.*—A chronic disease of the eye characterized by abrupt or insidious onset with inflammation of the conjunctivae and subepithelial infiltration, followed by granulation and pannus, by capillary infiltration of the cornea and by cicatrization leading to gross deformity of the eyelids, visual disability and possibly blindness.

Laboratory diagnosis is by finding cytoplasmic inclusion bodies, and by cytological changes in expressed follicular material.

A number of forms of chronic conjunctivitis of bacterial origin simulate trachoma and require differentiation.

2. *Etiologic agent.*—The virus of trachoma, one of the psittacosis-lymphogranuloma group.

3. *Source and reservoir of infection.*—Secretions from the eyes, and mucoid or purulent discharges of nasal mucous membranes of infected persons; tears of such persons also carry the infection.

4. *Mode of transmission.*—By direct contact with secretions of infected persons or by indirect contact with materials recently soiled therewith. Flies are vectors in Eastern countries. Carriers have not been demonstrated.

5. *Incubation period.*—Five to 12 days as determined by human volunteer experiments.

6. *Period of communicability.*—While active lesions are present in the conjunctivae and in the adnexed mucous membranes. After cicatrization is complete, communicability no longer exists, but reactivation of the disease may occur with reappearance of infective discharges.

7. *Susceptibility and resistance.*—Susceptibility is general; in all races, affects children more frequently than adults, and females more than males; particularly, persons of unclean habits and those whose eyes are irritated by exposure to sun, wind, and sand. Natural or acquired immunity has not been demonstrated.

8. *Occurrence.*—Worldwide, but with unequal and varying distribution in different countries and continental areas. High prevalence is generally associated with poor hygiene, poor nutrition and crowded living conditions, particularly in dry, dusty areas.

9. *Methods of control:*

A. Preventive measures:

1. In areas where trachoma is prevalent, careful and systematic examination of the eyes of children, especially school children.

2. The use in common of toilet articles and towels should be prohibited.

B. Control of the infected individual, contacts and environment:

1. Report to local health authority: Case report required in most states and countries, Class 2B (p. 7).

2. Isolation: Children should be excluded from school when active lesions exist and when adequate preventive measures are not practicable. With proper instruction of patient and family in means of preventing spread, and with adequate treatment of the patient, no need exists for isolation.

3. Concurrent disinfection: Of eye discharges and articles soiled therewith.

4. Terminal disinfection: None.

5. Quarantine: None.

6. Immunization: None.

7. Investigation of contacts and source of infection: Members of the family, playmates and schoolmates.

8. Specific treatment: Sulfonamides orally, an initial loading dose and smaller amounts thereafter for about 20 days. After an interval without treatment, the course is repeated. Sulfonamides are also used locally. Recent reports indicate the tetracycline antibiotics or chloramphenicol are equally effective.

C. Epidemic measures: None.

D. International measures: None.

TRICHINOSIS

1. *Identification.*—An infection arising through invasion of human and animal hosts by larvae (trichinae) of a parasitic nematode, Trichinella spiralis. Clinical disease in man is markedly irregular, severity varying with number of trichinae invading, tissue invaded and physiological state of the host. Sudden appearance of edema of upper eyelids is a common, early, and characteristic sign of clinical trichinosis, usually about the eleventh day of infection and sometimes followed by subconjunctival and retinal hemorrhage, pain and photophobia. Gastrointestinal symptoms may precede or accompany ocular manifestations. Muscle soreness and pain, skin lesions, thirst, profuse sweating, chills, weakness, prostration and rapidly increasing eosinophil count may shortly follow ocular signs. Fever is usual, remittent, and terminates by lysis after about a week; sometimes as much as 40° C. (104° F.) for several days. Respiratory and neurological symptoms may appear in the third to sixth week. Myocardial failure, when it occurs, is between the fourth and eighth weeks. Trichinosis is usually a mild febrile disease.

Daily study of blood smears for increasing eosinophilia is the most useful diagnostic laboratory procedure. Skin tests, flocculation tests and complement fixation tests may aid diagnosis but are not in themselves conclusive. Search for parasites in feces, blood, spinal fluid and biopsied striated muscle is often futile.

2. *Etiologic agent.*—Trichinella spiralis.

3. *Source and reservoir of infection.*—The source of infection is meat of infected animals, chiefly pork and pork products, occasionally wild game. Swine and many wild animals, fox, wolf, bear, polar bear, marine mammals and rats are reservoirs of infection.

4. *Mode of transmission.*—Consumption of flesh of animals containing viable trichinae.

5. *Incubation period.*—Onset about 9 days after ingestion of infective meat with variations between 2 and 28 days.

6. *Period of communicability.*—Not directly transmitted in nature from man to man.

7. *Susceptibility and resistance.*—Susceptibility is general. Neither natural nor acquired immunity is known to occur in man; has been demonstrated in experimental animals.

8. *Occurrence.*—World-wide, but rare or absent in native populations of the tropics or where swine are fed on root vegetables, as in France. The parasite is particularly widespread in the United States, about one in every six necropsies showing infection; less prevalent in Canada and Mexico. The former high prevalence in Germany, Spain, Hungary and the lower Danube countries is now far less. Clinical cases occur more frequently than indicated by morbidity reports; often confused with other illnesses and patients with mild infection do not seek medical aid. No selection by age, sex, race, region, season, or climate except as these affect the eating of insufficiently cooked flesh of infected hogs.

9. *Methods of control:*

A. Preventive measures:

1. Inauguration of local and state meat inspection to assure adequate processing of all pork products not under federal inspection and customarily eaten without further adequate cooking by the consumer.

2. Encouragement of farmers and hog raisers in the use of standard swine sanitation practices which will reduce opportunity for trichinal infection in swine, such as burial or other adequate disposal of swine and rat carcasses to prevent hogs from feeding on them; burning, burial, or other adequate disposal of swine offal so that swine or rats do not eat it; control of rats, particularly on farms and around hog-raising establishments and stockyards; rats probably constitute a minor source of swine trichinosis.

3. Elimination of the current practice of feeding uncooked garbage and offal to swine and the adoption and enforcement of suitable laws and regulations ensuring cooking such material before its consumption by swine. In Great Britain and Canada it is illegal to feed unboiled swill to swine.

4. Cooking of all fresh pork and pork products by the consumer at a temperature and for a time sufficient to allow all parts of the meat to reach at least 65.6° C. (150° F.) (a temperature which allows a good margin of safety) unless established that these meat products have been processed under federal or other official regulations adequate for the destruction of trichinae.

5. Low temperatures maintained in central portions of pork, are believed effective in killing trichina larvae; such as − 27° C. (− 16° F.) for 36 hours. Storage in home freezers as a safeguard against trichinosis is not to be depended upon.

B. Control of the infected individual, contacts and environment:
1. Report to local health authority: Case report desirably required in most states and countries, Class 2B (p. 7).
2. Isolation: None.
3. Concurrent disinfection: None.
4. Terminal disinfection: None.
5. Quarantine: None.
6. Immunization: None.
7. Investigation of contacts and source of infection: More likely a community than a case effort.
8. Specific treatment: None.

C. Epidemic measures: Establish the diagnosis. Examine dietary histories and institute epidemiologic study to determine the common food involved. Destroy remainders of food and initiate measures to correct faulty practices responsible.

D. International measures: None.

TRICHOMONIASIS

1. *Identification.*—A common non-fatal infection of the genito-urinary tract characterized in women by vaginitis associated with profuse leukorrhea and thin, foamy, yellowish discharge of foul odor. The vaginal mucosa is inflamed, frequently with small petechial punctate hemorrhagic lesions. In men, the infectious agent lives in the prostate urethra, or prepuce, rarely producing symptoms or demonstrable lesion.

Diagnosis is through identification of the motile parasite by direct and immediate microscopic examination of discharges.

2. *Etiologic agent.*—Trichomonas vaginalis, a protozoan.

3. *Source and reservoir of infection.*—Vaginal and urethral discharges of infected persons.

4. *Mode of transmission.*—By sexual intercourse with infected persons; possibly by contact with contaminated articles.

5. *Incubation period.*—Four to twenty days, average seven days.

6. *Period of communicability.*—For the duration of the infection.

7. *Susceptibility and resistance.*—General and high grade susceptibility to infection but clinical disease is mainly in females.

8. *Occurrence.*—In selected areas of the United States the incidence among Negroes is twice that of whites. Geographically wide spread, and a frequent disease of all continents and all peoples, primarily of adults, with highest incidence among young girls and women, aged 16 to 35 years.

9. *Methods of control:*

   A. Preventive measures:

      1. Avoidance of sexual intercourse with known infected individuals.

      2. Rigid personal hygiene in the use of public toilet facilities.

   B. Control of the infected individual, contacts and environment:

      1. Report to local health authority: Official report not ordinarily justifiable, Class 5 (p. 7).

      2. Isolation: None; avoid sexual relations during period of infection and treatment.

      3. Concurrent disinfection: None; the organisms can not withstand drying.

      4. Terminal disinfection: None.

      5. Quarantine: None.

      6. Immunization: None.

      7. Investigation of contacts and source of infection: Marital partner, particularly if a recurrent infection.

      8. Specific treatment: Most infected females respond promptly to chemotherapy with acetarsone, silver picrate or diodoquin.

   C. Epidemic measures: None.

   D. International measures: None.

TRICHURIASIS

1. *Identification.*—A nematode infection of the large intestine. Light infections are often asymptomatic and detected only when fecal examination reveals eggs. With heavy infections, intermittent abdominal discomfort, most commonly localized in the right lower quadrant, diarrhea, emaciation and anemia are observed. Synonyms: Trichocephaliasis, Whipworm Disease.

   Diagnosis of infection is by demonstration of eggs in the feces.

2. *Etiologic agent.*—Trichuris trichiura (Trichocephalus trichiurus), the human whipworm.

3. *Source and reservoir of infection.*—Feces of infected persons containing eggs of the parasite.

4. *Mode of transmission.*—Indirect, in that eggs passed in feces require at least ten days outside the body for embryonation in the soil. Ingestion of fully embryonated eggs derived from soil contaminated with human feces is followed by hatching and attachment of the developing worm to the mucosa of the cecum and proximal colon.

5. *Incubation period.*—From ingestion of eggs to passage of eggs, about 90 days; the incubation period, until symptoms appear, is longer, variable and indefinite.

6. *Period of communicability.*—As long as eggs are passed in feces

7. *Susceptibility and resistance.*—Susceptibility is general.

8. *Occurrence.*—Cosmopolitan, especially in warm, moist regions.

9. *Methods of control:*

   A. Preventive measures:

   1. Provision of adequate facilities for proper disposal of feces and prevention of soil contamination in areas immediately adjacent to houses, particularly in play areas of children.

   2. In rural areas, privies should be so constructed as to obviate dissemination of eggs through overflow, drainage or similar circumstance.

   3. Education of all members of the family, particularly children, to use toilet facilities.

   4. Encouragement of satisfactory hygienic habits on the part of children, especially the practice of washing the hands before handling food.

   B. Control of the infected individual, contacts and environment:

   1. Report to local health authority: Official report not ordinarily justifiable, Class 5 (p. 7). School health authorities should be advised of unusual prevalence in school populations.

   2. Isolation: None.

   3. Concurrent disinfection: None; sanitary disposal of feces.

   4. Terminal disinfection: None.

   5. Quarantine: None.

   6. Immunization: None.

   7. Investigation of contacts and source of infection: Fecal examination of members of family group, especially children, and of playmates.

   8. Specific treatment: No known effective chemotherapy; retention enemas of hexylresorcinol are partially effective.

   C. Epidemic measures: Not applicable.

   D. International measures: None.

TRYPANOSOMIASIS, AFRICAN

1. *Identification.*—A protozoan disease confined to tropical Africa, characterized in its early stage by fever, intense headache, insomnia, lymph node enlargement (especially posterior cervical), anemia, local edema and rash; and in its later stages by wasting, somnolence and other symptoms due to involvement of the central nervous system. The disease may run a protracted course of several years, or be rapidly fatal within a few months; a highly fatal disease. Synonym: African Sleeping Sickness.

   Definitive diagnosis in early stages is by finding trypanosomes in the peripheral blood or by lymph node puncture; in late stages, in the cerebrospinal fluid. Inoculation of rats, guinea pigs or monkeys with blood or lymph, or culture on appropriate media, are also used.

2. *Etiologic agent.*—Trypanosoma gambiense and T. rhodesiense, both probably varieties of the same species, T. brucei.

3. *Source and reservoir of infection.*—Immediate source is infected tsetse fly. Reservoirs of both gambiense and rhodesiense are the blood of infected persons. Wild game, especially antelopes, and domestic cattle and pigs are the chief animal reservoirs, and may occasionally be the source of human infection.

4. *Mode of transmission.*—By the bite of certain species of Glossina, tsetse flies. Four species are mainly concerned, G. palpalis, G. tachinoides, G. morsitans, and G. swynnertoni. In nature, the first two transmit T. gambiense and the latter two T. rhodesiense infections, although in the laboratory many other species are capable of transmitting both infections. The fly is infected by biting an infected person or animal. The parasite develops in the gut and proventriculus of the fly, the cycle requiring 18 days or longer according to temperature and other factors. Infection is conveyed by the bite. The metacyclic forms are injected with the salivary gland secretion into the wound made by the proboscis of the fly. Direct mechanical transmission by blood on proboscis of glossina is presumably possible. Once infected, a tsetse fly remains infective for life, up to 3 months; infection is not passed from generation to generation. A few cases of congenital infection in man have been reported.

5. *Incubation period.*—Usually 2 to 3 weeks. May be as short as 7 days.

6. *Period of communicability.*—As long as the parasite exists in the blood of the infected person; extremely variable in untreated cases; in late as well as in early stages of the disease.

7. *Susceptibility and resistance.*—Susceptibility is general, but the African native shows greater resistance than the European, in whom the disease tends to run a more acute course. Some patients recover without symptoms of central nervous system involvement; inapparent infection is known.

8. *Occurrence.*—The disease is confined to tropical Africa between 15° N. and 20° S., corresponding to distribution of the tsetse fly. A prevalence of 30 percent of a population has been demonstrated in some regions. Epidemics tend to occur when the disease is introduced into non-immune populations. In regions where G. palpalis is the principal vector, infection occurs mainly along streams (Gambia, Liberia, Sierra Leone, Gold Coast, Congo, Sudan, Uganda). Where G. morsitans is the principal vector, infection is over wider dry areas (Mosambique, Nyasaland, Rhodesia, Tanganyika).

9. *Methods of control:*

   A. Preventive measures:

   1. Mass treatment of whole local populations with appropriate chemotherapeutic agents in order to lower index of new infections.
   2. Wide and if necessary repeated clearings of bush around villages, along lines of communication, especially streams, near houses and roads. More likely to be successful against G. palpalis than other species.
   3. A concentration of the population in relatively large villages.
   4. Fly control by all practicable means including use of insecticides with residual effect, trapping, flypaper, and handnets.
   5. Destruction of pupae in breeding places.

6. Segregation of big game into game reserves away from human habitation (for G. morsitans).

7. Education of the population as to the mode of spread and methods of prevention.

8. Individual protection can be achieved temporarily by administration of an appropriate chemoprophylactic agent, preferably pentamidine, a single adult dose 250 mgm. intramuscularly, which protects for about six months.

B. Control of the infected individual, contacts and environment:

1. Report to local health authority: In selected endemic areas to obtain records of prevalence and to encourage control measures; not a reportable disease in most countries, Class 3B (p. 7).

2. Isolation: Patients with trypanosomes in the blood should be protected from bites of tsetse flies; isolation not practicable. Legal restrictions are placed on movement of untreated patients in some countries.

3. Concurrent disinfection: None.

4. Terminal disinfection: None.

5. Quarantine: None.

6. Immunization: None.

7. Investigation of contacts and source of infection: Should be done in connection with study of infected population groups.

8. Specific treatment: Rhodesiense infection is much more resistant than gambiense to chemotherapy. Before the nervous system is involved, Bayer 205 (antrypol suramin) is used intravenously for both T. gambiense and T. rhodesiense infection.

Tryparsamide is indicated in late T. gambiense infections. Serious side effects are possible; interrupt treatment if visual disturbances appear. Various combinations of Bayer 205 and tryparsamide are used for possible synergic effect. Melarsen and its derivatives may be useful in tryparsamide-resistant T. gambiense infections. Prognosis in advanced T. rhodesiense infection is poor with all treatment; Mel B and arsobal have been used recently with good effect in both gambiense and rhodesiense infections.

Pentamidine is effective in early T. gambiense infections, and is practically non-toxic; may be combined with tryparsamide; has not replaced Bayer 205 in treatment of T. rhodesiense infections.

C. Epidemic measures: In presence of an epidemic or in localized areas of high incidence, it may be necessary to move villages from sources of infection to fly-free areas. Other measures as in 9A.

D. International measures: Cooperative efforts of governments in endemic areas should be promoted. An International Bureau for Trypanosomiasis, acting as a clearing center for information, exists in Brazzaville, French Equatorial Africa.

TRYPANOSOMIASIS, AMERICAN

1. *Identification.*—A protozoan disease in which the parasite exists in the peripheral blood in the trypanosome form and in muscle and other tissues as leishmania-form bodies. The acute stage, lasting several weeks, is characterized by fever, malaise, enlargement of spleen and liver, and myocardial damage. Other early physical signs are unilateral edema of the eyelids extending to the face with red-purple discoloration of the skin, inflammation and swelling of the lachrymal glands, conjunctivitis and regional lymphadenopathy. The disease may become chronic with encephalopathy or end with gradual myocardial failure; death is uncommon. Many infected persons, especially adults, have few or no clinical manifestations. Synonym: Enfermedad de Chagas.

   Definitive diagnosis is by finding trypanosome forms in the peripheral blood during febrile episodes, or leishmania forms by muscle biopsy; by culture, by inoculation of albino rats, or by xenodiagnosis (feeding non-infected triatomine bugs on the patient and finding characteristic trypanosomes in the gut). A complement fixation test provides presumptive evidence.

   Two other species of trypanosome, T. rangeli and T. ariarii, have been found in blood films of man in Guatemala, Venezuela and Colombia; their distribution in other countries is unknown. They produce no demonstrable clinical disease, and are distinguishable from T. cruzi by morphological criteria.

2. *Etiologic agent.*—Trypanosoma cruzi, a hemoflagellate.

3. *Source and reservoir of infection.*—Source of infection is a bug; reservoirs include infected persons and a number of domestic and wild animals, such as dogs, cats, wood rats, opossums, and armadillos.

4. *Mode of transmission.*—By the fecal material of infected insect vectors; various blood sucking species of Reduviidae (cone-nosed bugs), especially of Triatoma, Rhodnius and Panstrongylus which frequently attack man. Infection may take place through conjunctivae, mucous membranes, abrasions, or wounds in the skin. Probably not transmitted by the actual act of biting; transmission by blood tranfusion has been noted.

5. *Incubation period.*—About 7 to 14 days.

6. *Period of communicability.*—Not directly communicable in nature from man to man; organisms are present in the blood only during the acute, febrile period.

7. *Susceptibility and resistance.*—Children, especially infants under 2 years of age, are particularly susceptible.

8. *Occurrence.*—The disease has a wide geographic distribution in Central and South America and is highly endemic in some areas. Cases have been found in southern Mexico. No natural infection of man has been reported in the United States but several species of Triatoma have been shown to be carriers of Trypanosoma cruzi in Texas, New Mexico, Arizona, and California, and wild rodents and opossums have been found infected in these areas.

9. *Methods of control:*

   A. Preventive measures:

      1. Construction or repair of dwellings so that they do not afford hiding places for the insect vector or shelter for the wild hosts.

194

2. Elimination of infected domestic animals and destruction of the habitations of the wild hosts in known endemic areas.
3. Use of a bed net in houses infested by the vector.
4. Systematic attack upon vectors through use of effective insecticides, especially those having residual action, with hexachlorocyclohexane much used in endemic areas.

B. Control of the infected individual, contacts and environment:

1. Report to local health authority: In selected endemic areas; not a reportable disease in most countries, Class 3B (p. 7).
2. Isolation: None.
3. Concurrent disinfection: None.
4. Terminal disinfection: None.
5. Quarantine: None.
6. Immunization: None.
7. Investigation of contacts and source of infection: Search of bedding and rooms for the vector, and investigation among domestic and wild animals for evidence of infection. Other members of the family should be examined for evidence of infection.
8. Specific treatment: Bayer 7602 (Ac), a 4-aminoquinoline, gives good results in some cases and has little or no effect in others. Tryparsamide and suramin are ineffective.

C. Epidemic measures: In areas of high incidence, field surveys to determine distribution and frequency of vectors.

D. International measures: None.

TUBERCULOSIS

1. *Identification.*—A chronic bacterial disease of great importance as a cause of death in nearly all parts of the world. Primary infection usually goes unnoticed clinically; some patients have fever, vague constitutional symptoms, or roentgenographic evidence of infiltration of the lungs and enlarged tracheobronchial nodes. The course of events thereafter is subject to much variation. Pleurisy with effusion may occur; in some areas, notably the Scandinavian countries, erythema nodosum is common. Some few individuals develop disseminated tuberculosis. Such developments are more likely within the first 6 to 12 months. Usually, however, the lesions heal spontaneously, leaving no residual changes except tuberculin sensitivity and occasionally pulmonary or tracheobronchial node calcifications. Disseminated or extrapulmonary (particularly skeletal) tuberculosis develops more often in infants and in Negroes. In late childhood primary disease is likely to be benign, and in young adults, it may resemble, or merge into pulmonary tuberculosis.

Pulmonary tuberculosis characteristically has a chronic variable course, with exacerbations and remissions but capable of arrest at any stage. Three stages (minimal, moderately advanced and far advanced) are distinguished according to extent of lung involvement; activity is determined by progression or retrogression as detected in serial roentgenograms, by presence of tubercle bacilli, and by symptoms. Abnormal roentgen shadows indicative of pulmonary infiltration, excavation, or fibrosis are common in advance of clinical manifestations. Symptoms of cough, fatigue, fever, weight loss, hoarseness, chest pain and hemoptysis and physical signs of dullness and rales are usual features of advanced disease.

Specific diagnosis is by demonstration of tubercle bacilli in sputum by stained smear, concentration and culture, or animal inoculation. Negative results on microscopic examination of sputum do not rule out tuberculosis; repeated examinations with more sensitive methods are eventually successful in most active cases; gastric washings or laryngeal swabs may be examined where sputum is absent or negative. Tuberculin test is positive in active tuberculosis except in critically ill persons; a negative reaction aids differential diagnosis.

Extrapulmonary tuberculosis is an early or late result of hematogenous dissemination of tubercle bacilli during the primary phase, as miliary tuberculosis, tuberculosis of bones and joints, central nervous system (tuberculous meningitis), lymphatic glands, and kidneys; or as a complication of pulmonary tuberculosis, involving intestines or larynx. Diagnosis is by isolation of tubercle bacilli from a lesion or exudate (cerebrospinal fluid in meningitis) or by histopathology. In the United States these forms are far less common than pulmonary tuberculosis, and as causes of death are decreasing more rapidly.

2. *Etiologic agent.*—Mycobacterium tuberculosis, tubercle bacillus. The human type causes nearly all pulmonary tuberculosis, the bovine type a considerable share of extrapulmonary disease, proportions varying according to opportunities for infection.

3. *Source and reservoir of infection.*—Respiratory secretions of persons with "open" (bacillary-positive) pulmonary tuberculosis; milk from tuberculous cattle. Patients with extrapulmonary tuberculosis are usually not sources of infection.

4. *Mode of transmission.*—Coughing or sneezing by patients with open pulmonary tuberculosis sets up a cloud of infectious material; minute particles may be inhaled directly or after settling and resuspension as dust. Direct and indirect contact are important; alimentary infection, as by contaminated eating and drinking utensils, is less so. Infection usually results from the continued and intimate exposure that characterizes household relationships; some susceptible family contacts avoid infection for long periods.

Bovine tuberculosis is transmitted by ingestion of unpasteurized milk or dairy products from tuberculous cows, by airborne infection in barns and by handling contaminated animal products.

5. *Incubation period.*—From infection to demonstrable primary phase lesions, about 4 to 6 weeks; from infection to progressive pulmonary or extrapulmonary tuberculosis may be years, with the first 6 to 12 months most hazardous.

6. *Period of communicability.*—As long as tubercle bacilli are being discharged by the patient. Commences when a lesion becomes open (discharges tubercle bacilli) and continues until healed or death occurs. Some patients remain sputum-positive intermittently for years. Degree of communicability depends upon the number of bacilli discharged and hygienic practices of the patient. Chemotherapy, collapse therapy, and pulmonary resection commonly shorten communicability.

7. *Susceptibility and resistance.*—Susceptibility is general; highest in children under 3 years, lowest from 3 to 12 years, and intermediate thereafter; greater in aboriginal races than in populations long exposed to the disease; in the undernourished, neglected, and fatigued more than in the well fed and well cared for. Especially prevalent among persons with silicosis or diabetes. The resistance conferred by healed primary infection is difficult to assess, but is not complete.

8. *Occurrence.*—Among the most common communicable diseases of man, endemic in practically all populations. In most western nations, incidence and mortality are declining. Age at first infection varies; persons living in cities ordinarily are infected earlier than in rural areas, and children living in household contact with a case are likely to be infected at a comparatively early age. Prevalence of infection and disease varies greatly in different areas; in some places a majority of adults are negative to usual doses of tuberculin. Photofluorographic surveys show prevalence of pulmonary tuberculosis to be low under age 15, rising gradually thereafter, although a large proportion of lesions of older persons are inactive. Prevalence of infection and roentgenographically demonstrable disease vary less with race than does mortality. In the United States, mortality is highest among infants and adult males beyond middle age. Mortality rates commonly reflect the social and economic welfare of a region; in many countries tuberculosis remains an important cause of death, with rates in excess of 100 per 100,000 population per year; in others rates are below 20. Reported cases in the United States show prevalence declining more slowly than mortality; this is attributable to improvements in case-finding, wider use of roentgenograms, and probably altered survivorship.

9. *Methods of control:*

    A. Preventive measures:

        1. Education of the public in the danger of tuberculosis, its mode of spread, and methods of control.

        2. Provision of adequate hospital facilities for isolation and treatment of active cases. The minimum number of beds needed per annual tuberculosis death is 2.5 in most communities of the United States.

        3. Provision of roentgenographic and clinical facilities for examination of contacts and suspects, and for clinical supervision and treatment of ambulant patients and those not hospitalized.

        4. Public health nursing service for home supervision of patients and to encourage and arrange for examination of contacts.

        5. Insuring a safe milk supply, through pasteurization of milk and elimination of tuberculosis among dairy cattle; meat inspection and condemning of all tuberculous carcasses.

        6. Measures to limit inhalation of dangerous concentrations of silica dust in industrial plants and mines.

        7. Routine roentgenographic examination of groups that have a higher prevalence of tuberculosis than the general population, such as nurses, medical students, patients and outpatients in general and mental hospitals, and selected groups of industrial workers; also those who constitute a special hazard to others if infected, to include pregnant women and school personnel.

8. Photofluorographic screening of adult populations where feasible; periodic resurveys should be made.

9. The role of BCG vaccination of uninfected persons is still unsettled. In many areas where mortality rates are high and economic resources do not permit a complete control program, mass vaccination of uninfected children and young adults is practiced, but its efficacy is still under evaluation. Vaccination has been advocated for newborn infants in communities with high morbidity, for household contacts of cases, for susceptible racial groups and for persons with unusual exposure by reason of occupation, such as medical and nursing students. In areas where mortality and morbidity from tuberculosis are low, and other control measures are available, the place of BCG vaccination in control of tuberculosis presently appears to be minor.

B. Control of the infected individual, contacts, and environment:

1. Report to local health authority: Obligatory case report in most states and countries, Class 2B (p. 7). Health departments should maintain a current register of active cases.

2. Isolation: A period of hospital or sanatorium treatment removes a focus of infection from the home, teaches the patient hygienic essentials of tuberculosis control, and increases the chances of recovery. Public health nursing supervision for patients remaining at home, including instruction in personal hygiene; compulsory isolation of those with open tuberculosis who do not observe necessary precautions is occasionally required.

3. Concurrent disinfection: Of sputum and articles soiled therewith, including handkerchiefs, cloths, or paper napkins, and of eating utensils used by patient. Patients should be trained to cover mouth and nose in coughing and sneezing.

4. Terminal disinfection: Cleaning. Wet cleaning of walls and floors and subsequent exposure to sunlight and fresh air.

5. Quarantine: None.

6. Immunization: BCG vaccination of tuberculin negative contacts may be warranted. See Section 9A9.

7. Investigation of contacts and source of infection: All members of the household of a newly discovered case and all intimate extra-household contacts should be examined roentgenologically, with particular attention to elderly persons with chronic cough. Annual retesting of tuberculin-negative persons, with intensive study of converters and their contacts, has been effective in some areas in disclosing early lesions, as well as finding previously unrecognized sources of infection.

8. Specific treatment: Most primary infections heal without treatment; if discovered in an active stage in susceptible age and racial groups, antimicrobial drug therapy may be instituted.

Active cases of pulmonary tuberculosis should be in a hospital, or on a hospital regimen of rest followed by graduated resumption of activity. Prompt treatment with antimicrobial drugs is indicated for most cases; choice of regimens is rapidly widening with increasing experience. At present a combination of streptomycin and para-aminosalicylic acid (PAS) is commonly employed in adults for six months to a year or more; toxic reactions are to be watched for and in vitro tests made for streptomycin resistance of tubercle bacilli isolated from the patient. Isoniazid is also effective, used alone or in combination with PAS, streptomycin or both. A combination of these three drugs is ordinarily reserved for serious situations, in order to avoid development of strains of tubercle bacilli resistant to one or the other of the drugs.

Reversible forms of lung collapse (pneumothorax, pneumoperitoneum and phrenic nerve interruption) are less frequently employed than formerly. Thoracoplasty is selectively indicated. Pulmonary resection to remove diseased lung is used increasingly, as well as the less radical procedure of extrapleural plombage.

In extrapulmonary tuberculosis, medical therapy as described above for pulmonary tuberculosis is combined with specific measures, often surgical, suited to the particular form and type of disease.

In miliary and meningeal tuberculosis, treatment should be started immediately with isoniazid by mouth, supplemented by intramuscular streptomycin. In comatose patients, streptomycin may also be given intrathecally. Therapy should be continued at least 6 months.

C. Epidemic measures:

1. Alertness to recognize the occasional cluster of new cases resulting from contacts with an unrecognized infectious case; intensive search for the source of infection in such situations.

D. International measures: Roentgenographic screening of individuals prior to emigration, to detect communicable and potentially communicable tuberculosis.

TULAREMIA

1. *Identification.*—An infectious disease of wild mammals and man; onset is sudden, with chills and fever, the patient usually prostrated and confined to bed. Lymph nodes draining the site of original infection become swollen and tender, and commonly suppurate. The fatality is about 5%.

Diagnosis is confirmed by inoculation of animals with material from local lesions or with sputum, by isolation of the microorganism bacteriologically and by agglutination reaction. Skin test is less reliable.

2. *Etiologic agent.*—Pasteurella tularensis (Bacterium tularense).

3. *Source and reservoir of infection.*—Many species of wild animals and some domesticated animals; wild rabbits and hares, woodchuck, coyote, muskrat, opossum, tree squirrel, quail, skunk, water rat of

Europe (Arvicola emphibus), cat, deer, dog, fox, hog, sage hen, sheep and bull snake; also woodticks.

4. *Mode of transmission.*—By bite of infected flies or ticks, and by inoculation of skin or conjunctival sac through handling infected animals, as in skinning, dressing, or performing necropsies, or by fluids from infected flies, ticks, rabbits, and woodchucks. Arthropods directly related to disease in man are the following: one species of deer fly, Chrysops discalis; the wood tick, Dermacentor andersoni; the dog tick, Dermacentor variabilis and the Lone Star tick, Amblyomma americanum; and in Sweden the mosquito, Aedes cinereus. Ingestion of insufficiently cooked rabbit meat and drinking contaminated water. Rare cases occur from bites of coyotes, skunks, hogs, cats, and dogs, where the mouth of the animal was presumably contaminated from eating infected rabbits. Laboratory infections are relatively frequent.

5. *Period of incubation.*—From 24 hours to 10 days, usually 3 days.

6. *Period of communicability.*—Not communicable from man to man. The infectious agent may be found in the blood of man during the first 2 weeks of the disease, and in lesions of the disease up to a month from onset and sometimes longer. Flies are infective for 14 days, ticks throughout their lifetime, about two years. Refrigerated rabbits kept constantly frozen at − 15° C. (5° F.) may remain infective for 3½ years.

7. *Susceptibility and resistance.*—All ages are susceptible; permanent immunity follows recovery. Through abrasion of the hand or by contact with contaminated material, an immune person may acquire a local tularemic papule which harbors virulent organisms but causes no notable constitutional reaction.

8. *Occurrence.*—Throughout North America, in many parts of continental Europe and in Japan; unknown in Australia. Occurs in the United States in every month of the year, but especially autumn during the rabbit hunting season.

9. *Methods of control:*

A. Preventive measures:

1. Avoid bites of flies and ticks or handling such arthropods when working in infected areas during seasonal incidence of bloodsucking flies and ticks.

2. The use of rubber gloves by persons engaged in dressing wild rabbits or in performing necropsies on infected laboratory animals will usually prevent occupational infections; employment of immune persons for dressing wild rabbits or conducting laboratory experiments. Thorough cooking of meat of wild rabbits.

3. Avoid drinking raw water in areas where the disease prevails among wild animals.

B. Control of the infected individual, contacts and environment:

1. Report to local health authority: In selected endemic areas (USA); in many countries not a reportable disease, Class 3A (p. 7).

2. Isolation: None.

3. Concurrent disinfection: Of discharges from ulcer, lymph nodes, or conjunctival sac.

4. Terminal disinfection: None.

5. Quarantine: None.
6. Immunization: None.
7. Investigation of contacts and source of infection: Should be undertaken in each case.
8. Specific treatment: Streptomycin, the tetracyclines and chloramphenicol are effective when continued until four to five days of normal temperature.

C. Epidemic measures: Search for sources of infection related to arthropods, to animal hosts and to water. Control measures as thus indicated (see 9A). Interstate or interarea shipment of infected animals or carcasses should be prohibited.

D. International measures: None.

TYPHOID FEVER

1. *Identification.*—A systemic infection characterized by continued fever, involvement of lymphoid tissues, especially ulceration of Peyer's patches, enlargement of spleen, rose spots on trunk, and diarrhea. Many mild, atypical infections are often unrecognized. A usual fatality of 10% is reduced to 2 to 3% by antibiotic therapy. Synonyms: Enteric Fever, Typhus Abdominalis.

Typhoid bacilli are found in blood during first two weeks and in feces and urine after second week. Widal reaction becomes positive during second week; O agglutinins more significant than H agglutinins.

2. *Etiologic agent.*—Salmonella typhosa, typhoid bacillus. About 30 types can be distinguished by Vi-phage.

3. *Source and reservoir of infection.*—Feces and urine of infected persons. Family contacts may be transient carriers; fecal carriers more common than urinary. The carrier state is most common among persons over 40 years of age, especially females; fecal carriers frequently have a typhoid cholecystitis, usually permanent unless cholecystectomy is done.

4. *Mode of transmission.*—Direct or indirect contact with patient or carrier. Principal vehicles of indirect spread are contaminated water and food. Raw fruits and vegetables are important factors in some parts of the world; milk, milk products and shellfish in others. Contamination is usually by hands of carrier or missed case. Under some conditions, flies are vectors.

5. *Incubation period.*—Variable; average 2 weeks, usual range 1 to 3 weeks.

6. *Period of communicability.*—As long as typhoid bacilli appear in excreta; usually from appearance of prodromal symptoms, throughout illness, and for varying period of time after cessation of symptoms. About 10% of patients will discharge bacilli three months after onset; 2 to 5% become permanent carriers.

7. *Susceptibility and resistance.*—Susceptibility is general, although many adults appear to acquire immunity through unrecognized infections; attack rates decline with age after second or third decades. A high degree of resistance usually follows recovery. The degree of artificial active immunity conferred by typhoid vaccine is uncertain.

8. *Occurrence.*—Widespread throughout world. Endemic in some rural areas of United States, but commonly occurring as sporadic cases and as small contact and carrier epidemics; steadily falling in incidence, particularly in urban areas. Still common in many countries of the Far East, Middle East, eastern Europe, Central and South America, and in Africa.

9. *Methods of control:*

A. Preventive measures:

1. Protection and purification of public water supplies; construction of safe private supplies.

2. Sanitary disposal of human excreta.

3. Boiling of milk or pasteurization of milk and dairy products, including cheese.

4. Limitation of collection and marketing of shellfish to those from approved sources.

5. Sanitary supervision of processing, preparation and serving of all foods, especially those that are eaten raw; special attention to provision and use of hand-washing facilities.

6. Fly control, control of fly breeding, and protection of foods against fly contamination by screening.

7. Immunization with a vaccine of high antigenicity. The protection conferred by vaccination is under reevaluation. Current practice is to vaccinate persons subjected to unusual exposure through occupation or travel, those living in areas of high endemic incidence, and institutional populations in which maintenance of sanitation is difficult. Periodic reinforcing injections are desirable, commonly once in three years.

8. Discovery and supervision of typhoid carriers; those of duration exceeding 1 year may be released from supervision and restriction of occupation (9A.9) only after 6 consecutive negative cultures of authenticated specimens of feces and urine taken 1 month apart. (cf. 9B.2) Cholecystectomy usually ends the carrier state.

9. Instruction of convalescents and chronic carriers in personal hygiene, particularly as to sanitary disposal of excreta, handwashing after defecation and before eating, and exclusion from acting as food handlers.

10. Education of general public and particularly of food handlers concerning sources of infection and modes of transmission.

B. Control of the infected individual, contacts and environment:

1. Report to local health authority: Obligatory case report in most states and countries, Class 2A (p. 7).

2. Isolation: In flyproof room. Hospital care desirable for patients who cannot command adequate sanitary environment and nursing care at home. Release from supervision by local health authority should be by not less than three negative cultures of feces and urine, at least 24 hours apart and not earlier than one month after onset; if any one of this series is positive, not less than 3 negative cultures at intervals of 1 month and within the succeeding year. (9A.8)

3. Concurrent disinfection: Of feces and urine and articles soiled therewith. In communities with modern and ade-

quate sewage disposal systems, feces and urine can be disposed of directly into sewer without preliminary disinfection.

4. Terminal disinfection: Cleaning.

5. Quarantine: Family contacts should not be employed as food handlers during period of contact nor before repeated negative feces and urine cultures are obtained.

6. Immunization: Administration of typhoid vaccine to family, household and nursing contacts who have been or may be exposed to cases or carriers.

7. Investigation of contacts and source of infection: Actual or probable source of infection of every case should be determined by search for common and individual sources, unreported cases and carriers, or contaminated food, water, milk or shellfish. Presence of agglutinins in blood of suspected carriers is suggestive of the carrier state. Organisms from patients and carriers should be typed by phage to determine cases of same type and therefore of presumed common origin.

8. Specific treatment: Chloramphenicol; an initial oral loading dose is followed by oral doses every six hours until temperature is normal, then in smaller doses for a total of 14 days.

C. Epidemic measures:

1. Intensive search for case or carrier who is source of infection.

2. Exclusion of suspected food.

3. Boiling of milk or pasteurization or exclusion of suspected milk supplies or other suspected foods on epidemiologic evidence, pending elimination of cause of contamination.

4. Chlorination under competent supervision of suspected water supply or its exclusion. All water used for drinking must be chlorinated or boiled before use.

D. International measures: Inoculation of international travellers with triple typhoid vaccine (TAB, typhoid, paratyphoid A, paratyphoid B) is advisable for travel in all areas except the United States, Canada, Great Britain and Northwest Europe if not protected through previous attack.

TYPHUS FEVER

A. Epidemic or Classical Typhus (Louse-Borne)

1. *Identification.*—A rickettsial disease with a history of great epidemics and a continued existence in numerous areas of the world. The onset is variable, often sudden and marked by headache, chills, fever, and general pains; a macular eruption appears on the 5th or 6th day, toxemia is usually pronounced and the disease terminates in rapid lysis after about 2 weeks of fever. In the absence of specific therapy the fatality varies from 10 to 40% in different epidemics and increases with age. Mild infections may occur with eruption evanescent or absent, especially in vaccinated persons.

A recrudesence of epidemic typhus fever may occur years after the primary attack (Brill's disease); it differs from the classical type in that it need not be associated with lousiness and is milder, with fewer complications and lower fatality. Synonym: Typhus Exanthematicus.

The Weil-Felix reaction with Proteus OX19 is usually positive with serums obtained after the 10th day, the complement fixation test a few days later.

2. *Etiologic agent.*—Rickettsia prowazeki, var. prowazeki.

3. *Source and reservoir of infection.*—The source of infection is lice infected by feeding on blood of man with the febrile disease. Man is the reservoir and responsible for maintaining the infection during inter-epidemic periods. Patients with recrudescent typhus (Brill's disease) can infect lice and probably serve as foci for new outbreaks in louse-infested communities.

4. *Mode of transmission.*—Infected body lice, Pediculus humanus, excrete rickettsiae in their feces and usually defecate at the time of feeding. Man is infected by rubbing feces or crushed lice into the wound made by the bite or into superficial abrasions of the skin. Inhalation of dried infective louse feces as dust from dirty clothes may account for some infections.

5. *Incubation period.*—From 6 to 15 days, commonly 12 days.

6. *Period of communicability.*—Patients are infective for lice during the febrile illness and possibly for 2 or 3 days after the temperature returns to normal. The living louse is infective as soon as it begins to pass rickettsiae in feces; earlier if crushed. Under favorable conditions, rickettsiae remain viable in the dead louse for weeks. Not communicable in nature from man to man.

7. *Susceptibility and resistance.*—Susceptibility is general. The disease in children and in vaccinated adults is mild and may go unrecognized. Attack usually confers permanent immunity.

8. *Occurrence.*—In most colder areas of the world where appreciable groups of people live under unhygienic conditions and are lousy. Endemic centers exist in mountainous regions of Mexico and Central and South America, the Balkans and Central and Eastern Europe, North Africa and mountainous areas of Central and South Africa, and most of Asia except the humid tropics. Prior to modern methods of control, epidemics were frequent among military and refugee populations and in areas suffering famine or war.

9. *Methods of control:*

    A. Preventive measures:

        1. Application by hand or power blower of residual insecticide powder (10% DDT or newer lousicides) at appropriate intervals to clothes and persons of populations living under conditions favoring lousiness. Lice are known to develop DDT resistance; lindane may be substituted as a dusting powder.

        2. Improvement of living conditions with provision for frequent bathing and washing of clothing.

        3. Individual prophylaxis of persons subject to unusual risk through insecticide applied at appropriate intervals to clothing by dusting or by impregnation; immunization.

B. Control of the infected individual, contacts, and environment:

1. Report to local health authority: Case report universally required by international regulation, Class 1 (p. 6).

2. Isolation: Not required after proper delousing of patient, clothing, living quarters and household contacts.

3. Concurrent disinfection: Appropriate insecticide powder applied to clothing and bedding of patient and contacts; treatment of hair for louse eggs (nits) with tested chemical agents.

4. Terminal disinfection: If death occurs before delousing, thorough application of insecticides to body and clothing.

5. Quarantine: Exposed lousy susceptibles should be quarantined for 15 days but may be released after application of insecticide with residual effect.

6. Immunization: Of all immediate contacts.

7. Investigation of contacts and source of infection: Every effort should be made to trace the source of infection to direct or indirect contact with a preceding case.

8. Specific treatment: The tetracyclines or chloramphenicol orally in a loading dose followed by daily doses until the patient becomes afebrile (usually 2 days) and for one additional day.

C. Epidemic measures:

1. Delousing: The most important measure for the rapid control of typhus, where reporting has been good and numbers of cases are small, is application of insecticides with residual effect to all contacts. Where infection is known to be widespread, systematic application of residual insecticide to all persons in the community is indicated.

2. Immunization: Of persons in contact with cases; vaccination may be offered to entire community. The usual vaccines contain rickettsiae grown in yolk sac of developing chick embryo and inactivated by formalin. The vaccine is administered in 2 doses, one week apart; re-inoculation with a single dose every 4 months where danger of typhus persists. For vaccinated persons the risk of infection is reduced, the course of the disease modified and the case fatality lowered.

D. International measures:

1. Telegraphic notification of WHO and of adjacent countries, by governments, of the existence of an epidemic of typhus fever.

2. Measures applicable to ships, aircraft and land transport arriving from typhus areas are specified by International Sanitary Regulations (WHO Techn. Rep. Ser., No. 41, Geneva, 1951).

3. International travellers may leave a typhus area without restraint after thorough application of insecticide with residual effect. Vaccination is recommended for all persons entering areas where typhus is present.

B. Murine Typhus (Flea-borne, Endemic)

1. *Identification.*—The clinical course resembles that of epidemic typhus but tends to be milder. The fatality for all ages is about 2%, with prognosis grave in older people.

   The Weil-Felix reaction is usually positive with Proteus OX19 after the 9th day; the complement fixation reaction a few days later. Differential diagnosis from louse-borne typhus is by serologic tests using rickettsial suspensions.

2. *Etiologic agent.*—Rickettsia prowazeki, var. typhi (Rickettsia mooseri).

3. *Source and reservoir of infection.*—Fleas, commonly Xenopsylla cheopis, infected from rats which are the reservoir, Rattus rattus and Rattus norvegicus. The rodent disease is maintained in nature by a rat-flea-rat cycle.

4. *Mode of transmission.*—Infected fleas excrete rickettsiae in feces, defecate after sucking blood, and contaminate the fresh skin wound. Inhalation of dried infected flea feces may account for an occasional case.

5. *Incubation period.*—From 6 to 14 days, commonly 12 days.

6. *Period of communicability.*—Not communicable in nature from man to man.

7. *Susceptibility and resistance.*—Susceptibility is general. One attack confers immunity, not always permanent. Murine typhus vaccine (similar to epidemic typhus vaccine) has had field trial but requires further evaluation.

8. *Occurrence.*—World wide in areas where men and rats occupy the same buildings. Five thousand cases in the United States in 1945, but numbers are markedly less in recent years. Highest attack rates are in Gulf and South Atlantic seaboard states, mainly during summer months when fleas are abundant. Changes in agricultural practices and increased rat populations of farms make the disease increasingly rural, replacing the former urban distribution centered around feed and grain stores.

9. *Methods of control:*

   A. Preventive measures:
   1. Application of insecticide powders with residual activity (10% DDT or other compounds) to rat runs, burrows, and harborages.
   2. Rodent control measures should be delayed until flea populations have been reduced by insecticides, to avoid temporary increase in cases.

   B. Control of the infected individual, contacts and environment:
   1. Report to local health authority: Case report obligatory in most states and countries, Class 2B (p. 7).
   2. Isolation: None.
   3. Concurrent disinfection: None.
   4. Terminal disinfection: None.
   5. Quarantine: None.
   6. Immunization: None for contacts.
   7. Investigation of contacts and source of infection: Search for rodents around premises or home of patient.
   8. Specific treatment: As for epidemic typhus.

C. Epidemic measures: In endemic areas with numerous cases, widespread use of DDT has markedly reduced the flea index of rats, and incidence of infection in rats and man. Inoculation with an inactivated R. mooseri vaccine may be useful for limited groups in hazardous occupations but the efficiency of specific therapy eliminates the need for general protection of populations.

D. International measures: None.

YAWS

1. *Identification.*—An acute and chronic relapsing non-venereal treponematosis characterized by hypertrophic, granulomatous or ulcerative destructive lesions of the skin, and by destructive and hypertrophic changes in bone. Two to 8 weeks after exposure, a primary lesion appears at the site of inoculation as an ulcer or granuloma ("mother yaw"). In several weeks to several months, and often before the initial lesion has healed, mild constitutional symptoms appear, with generalized eruption of papules and granulomatous nodules, often in successive crops and lasting from a few months to several years, eventually developing into typical frambesiaform lesions. Eruptions of soles of the feet ("crab yaws") are common in this and the tertiary stage. The tertiary stage develops after an intervening latency, sometimes a matter of years, with destructive or profilerative lesions of bone and joint, and destructive lesions of skin. Unlike venereal syphilis, seldom involves the central nervous system or viscera; rarely if ever fatal. Synonyms: Frambesia Tropica, Pian, Bouba, Parangi and many others.

   Serologic tests for syphilis are reactive with the same frequency in yaws as in syphilis, becoming positive during the primary stage, remaining positive during the secondary stage and tending toward non-reactivity after many years of latency, even without specific therapy.

2. *Etiologic agent.*—Treponema pertenue.

3. *Source and reservoir of infection.*—An infected person; surface and exudates of early skin lesions.

4. *Mode of transmission.*—Principally by direct household or other contact with infectious lesions; perhaps also by indirect contact with contaminated articles; some evidence of vector transmission by a minute fly, Hippelates pallipes; transmission in utero not established.

5. *Incubation period.*—From 2 weeks to 3 months; generally 3 to 6 weeks.

6. *Period of communicability.*—Variable; may extend intermittently over several years while relapsing moist lesions are present; treponemata are not usually found in late ulcerative lesions.

7. *Susceptibility and resistance.*—No clear evidence of natural or racial immunity but acquired resistance against homologous strains seems established; resistance against heterologous strains is not disproved. Resistance develops slowly; is relatively weak during the first months or years and may be overcome by large reinfecting doses; later becomes solid unless suppressed by early treatment. Super-

infection in late latency may be manifested by late ulcerative lesions.

8. *Occurrence.*—Widely and unevenly distributed; affected by many variables within the physical and social environment. Predominantly a childhood disease but occurs in later life; males outnumber females. Primarily a disease of rural peoples of the tropics and subtropics; the lowest social and economic groups have the highest rates. Particularly common in equatorial Africa, the Caribbean area, parts of India, Ceylon, the Philippines, Burma, Indochina, Indonesia, Thailand and throughout the South Pacific Islands; endemic foci in parts of Brazil, Colombia, Venezuela and the Guianas and in several countries of Central America; sporadic cases occur in North America and Europe from infection contracted elsewhere.

9. *Methods of control.*—Venereal syphilis has declined significantly in many areas; the non-venereal treponematoses are a continuing problem. The etiologic agents of all these disorders are morphologically and biologically almost identical and the clinical syndromes produced are the result of epidemiologic rather than biologic differences.

A. Preventive measures: The following are applicable to yaws and to other non-venereal treponematoses.

1. General health promotional measures; health education, better sanitation and improved social and economic conditions over a period of years will lead to a lesser incidence.

2. In endemic areas education of the public about treponematosis; organization of intensive control activities on a community basis, to include analysis of the specific local problem, examination of entire populations, mass treatment of infected persons and contacts, and periodic assessment of results achieved.

3. Provision of facilities for early diagnosis and treatment on a continuing plan, whereby the mass control campaign (9A2 above) is eventually consolidated into permanent local health services providing early diagnosis and treatment to patients and contact investigation and health education to the community.

4. Emphasis on control of infectivity should not preclude treatment of disfiguring and incapacitating late manifestations nor the discovery and treatment of latent cases, since many late and latent lesions subsequently become reactivated and possibly infectious.

B. Control of the infected individual, contacts and environment:

1. Report to local health authority: In selected endemic areas; in many countries not a reportable disease, Class 3B (p. 7). Differentiation of venereal and non-venereal treponematoses with proper reporting of each has particular importance in evaluation of mass campaigns and in the consolidation period thereafter.

2. Isolation: None; avoid intimate personal contact until lesions are healed.

3. Concurrent disinfection: Care in disposal of discharges and articles contaminated therewith.

4. Terminal disinfection: None.

5. Quarantine: None.

6. Immunization: None.
7. Investigation of contacts and source of infection: All familial contacts should be treated, see 9B8 and 9C.
8. Specific treatment: Penicillin; for early infectious lesions in adults no less than 1.2 million units of procaine penicillin in oil with 2% aluminum monostearate, proportionately less for children, in one injection; the preventive dose for contacts is not less than half that for early infectious cases.

C. Epidemic measures: At the present time most control activities have to do with hyperendemic situations. The problem is broader than the control of the infected individual and his immediate contacts. In areas of high incidence a broad segment of the population at risk should be given a full course of antibiotic treatment in order to prevent or abort the disease, especially children of preschool and school age, where attack rates are commonly high. In areas of lower incidence such treatment may be restricted to intimate contacts (household and extra-household) regardless of age.

D. International measures:
1. Appropriate examination of groups of adolescents and young adults moving from areas of high prevalence of treponemal infections.

YELLOW FEVER

1. *Identification.*—An acute infectious disease of short duration and varying severity. The mildest cases are clinically indeterminate; typical attacks are characterized by sudden onset, fever, headache, backache, prostration, nausea and vomiting. As the disease progresses, the pulse rate slows in relation to temperature and albuminuria is pronounced. Leucopenia appears early, most pronounced about the fifth day. Common hemorrhagic symptoms include epistaxis, buccal bleeding, hematemesis and melena. Jaundice is moderate but postmortem icterus may be pronounced. The fatality among indigenous populations of endemic regions is less than 5 per cent; for persons of other origin, rates of 30 to 40% are common.

Laboratory procedures in diagnosis are isolation of virus from blood through animal inoculation; demonstration of antibodies in convalescent serum when absent during the first 4 days; and demonstration of typical histopathological lesions of the liver.

2. *Etiologic agent.*—The virus of yellow fever.

3. *Source and reservoir of infection.*—The immediate source of infection for man is an infected mosquito; in urban areas the reservoir of infection is an infected person; in forest areas, also man but mainly monkeys, marmosets and probably marsupials.

4. *Mode of transmission.*—In urban and certain rural areas, by the bite of the mosquito, Aëdes aegypti. In the forests of South America by the bite of forest mosquitoes that include Haemagogus spegazzinii, H. spegazzinii falco, H. capricornii, and Aëdes leucocelaenus. In East Africa, rural and sylvan transmission occurs through the

bite of Aëdes simpsoni, A. africanus, and possibly other Aëdes mosquitoes.

5. *Incubation period.*—Three to six days.

6. *Period of communicability.*—Shortly prior to onset of fever and for the first three days of illness. Highly communicable where many susceptible persons and abundant vector mosquitoes co-exist. Not communicable by contact or by fomites. The extrinsic incubation period of Aëdes aegypti varies with temperature, commonly 10 to 14 days, after which the mosquito is infective; mosquitoes once infected remain so for life.

7. *Susceptibility and resistance.*—Recovery from yellow fever is regularly followed by lasting immunity; second attacks are unknown. Mild, inapparent infections are common in endemic areas. Transient passive immunity in infants born to immune mothers may persist up to six months. In natural infection, antibodies appear in the blood within the first week. Active immunity is induced by inoculation with a suitable vaccine, see 9A3.

8. *Occurrence.*—All ages are susceptible; in endemic areas of urban yellow fever with many adults immune, more than half of cases are among children, the ratio of males to females being approximately equal. Jungle yellow fever of tropical America is predominantly a disease of adult males, with the 20 to 40 year age group most affected. Seasonal incidence follows rainfall and prevalence of local vector mosquitoes; commonest in summer months. In Colombia and part of Brazil the seasonal curve of jungle yellow fever is bi-modal. Geographic distribution of urban yellow fever has changed greatly as a result of mosquito control campaigns. In the Americas as a whole, the last case known to be transmitted by Aëdes aegypti was in Trinidad in 1954. Outbreaks of urban yellow fever are still reported from Africa. Available evidence indicates that jungle yellow fever is present from time to time in all countries of the mainland of the Americas, from Mexico south to Central and South America, with the exception of Uruguay and Chile where there are no tropical or subtropical forests with monkeys or other susceptible animals.

9. *Methods of control:*

A. Preventive measures:

    1. Control of Aëdes aegypti breeding is the most important factor in prevention of urban outbreaks of yellow fever and should be undertaken in towns and cities of countries where the disease is endemic. Complete control of urban yellow fever is possible in the Americas since A. aegypti is not a forest mosquito. Permanent protection is not to be had without a permanent control service.

    2. Sylvan or jungle yellow fever, transmitted by forest species of Aëdes and Haemagogus, cannot be controlled by any known anti-mosquito measures. Intensive vaccination programs are effective, particularly when aimed at persons living in rural areas whose daily occupation brings them into forests in yellow fever areas.

    3. Active immunization of all persons necessarily exposed to infection because of residence or occupation is necessary. Two living modified vaccines have had wide acceptance. The one (17-D strain) produces satisfactory immunity

after one inoculation. Antibodies appear from 7 to 10 days after vaccination and persist for at least 6 years, probably longer. A vaccine extensively used in West Africa combines living neurotropic yellow fever virus with vaccinia virus, applied once by scarification; effective, but reactions are more frequent and encephalitis is an occasional complication.

B. Control of the infected individual, contacts and environment:

1. Report to local health authority: Case report universally required by International Sanitary Regulation, Class 1 (p. 6).

2. Isolation: None; prevent access of mosquitoes to patient during first three days by screened sickroom or by spraying quarters with insecticide having residual effect.

3. Concurrent disinfection: None; home of patient and all houses in vicinity should be sprayed promptly with an insecticide having residual action, such as 5% DDT, benzene hexachloride or chlordane.

4. Terminal disinfection: None.

5. Quarantine: None.

6. Immunization: Family contacts and neighbors of patient not previously immunized should be vaccinated promptly.

7. Investigation of contacts and source of infection: Inquiry about areas of forest visited by patient 3 to 6 days before onset, to identify foci of jungle yellow fever; observation of all others visiting that tract of forest. Search of premises and place of work for mosquitoes believed capable of transmitting infection. Attention to mild febrile illnesses and unexplained deaths suggesting yellow fever.

8. Specific treatment: None.

C. Epidemic measures:

1. Urban or Aëdes aegypti transmitted yellow fever:

   a. Spray interior of all homes in community with residual insecticide, such as DDT or benzene hexachloride.

   b. Application of a larvicide to all water containers of the community; 2% DDT in ethyl alcohol has been used successfully in jars and barrels containing drinking water.

   c. Mass vaccination.

2. Jungle or sylvan yellow fever:

   a. Vaccination of all persons living near forested areas or entering forests.

   b. Avoidance of forests by unvaccinated individuals, and by vaccinated persons for the first week after vaccination; particularly those tracts of forest where infection has been localized.

3. In regions where yellow fever may occur, a viscerotome service should be organized to collect for diagnostic purposes small specimens of liver tissue from fatal febrile illnesses of ten days' duration or less; many cases and outbreaks otherwise missed are thereby discovered.

4. Immunity surveys by neutralization test, of human populations and of primates captured in forested areas, are useful in definite endemic areas.

D. International measures:

1. Telegraphic notification of WHO and of adjacent countries, by governments, of the existence of an epidemic of yellow fever.

2. Measures applicable to ships, aircraft and land transport arriving from yellow fever areas are specified in International Sanitary Regulations (WHO Techn. Rep. Ser. No. 41, Geneva, 1951).

3. Animal quarantine: Quarantine of monkeys and marmosets arriving from yellow fever areas may be required until seven days have elapsed after leaving.

4. International travellers: A valid anti-yellow fever vaccination certificate is required by most countries for travellers into or coming from recognized yellow fever zones of Africa and South America; otherwise, quarantine measures are applicable. The international certificate of vaccination is valid from 10 days after date of vaccination and for 6 years; if revaccinated within that time, from date of that revaccination and for 6 years.

INDEX

213